Caregivers:
Angels without Wings

Caregivers:
Angels without Wings

Peg Crandall

iUniverse, Inc.
New York Lincoln Shanghai

Caregivers: Angels without Wings

iUniverse, Inc.

For information address:
iUniverse, Inc.
2021 Pine Lake Road, Suite 100
Lincoln, NE 68512
www.iuniverse.com

ISBN: 0-595-32660-9

Printed in the United States of America

To my sister, Linda Trost, who has been our mother's primary caregiver for many years.

Contents

Foreword

Dear Caregivers:

I could not let *Caregivers: Angels without Wings* go to press without sharing a little something about its author. Peg Crandall is my older sister. For as long as I can remember, she has always been there for me.

When she came home from college on weekends, she always set aside a few hours to do something special with her little sister. Just the two of us. Dinner at the airport (that was when the airport was a very special place) or renting a canoe on the lake in Forest Park. How "cool" I thought it was to be out with someone ten years older than me.

She was there the day I ran home from school, certain I was going to bleed to death. She was the one who explained what it meant to "become a woman" as she walked me around and around the dining room table, assuring me that exercise would help relieve the cramps. When I had breast cancer, who cried with me, laughed with me, and talked with me? My big sister and caregiver. When Peg told me she had breast cancer I felt responsible. As always, she talked me through my feelings, not worrying about hers. As I proceeded through my divorce, she was there to listen, never judging.

Peg and I have lived at least 800 miles apart for forty-five years and yet she is always there for me. I recently had major surgery. Naturally, who came to help me after I was released from the hospital? Peg and her husband Marv. They cooked, cleaned, chauffeured, and entertained. Marv even completed numerous chores I had on a "honey-do" list.

There is something I would like for caregivers to know. The person you are caring for will never be able to fully express their gratitude for your acts of kindness. Even your simple gestures such as sending a card, giving a tray of rice krispies treats (my particular favorite), or stopping by to visit, means so much.

The most important thing for caregivers to understand is that doctors can help heal our bodies but caregivers (and sisters) heal our souls. We could not make it without the care we receive from our family and friends.

I have very much enjoyed sharing the adventure Peg experienced as she wrote *Caregivers: Angels without Wings*. She is a caregiver. I hope you gain support as you read her book.

With sincere gratitude for all caregivers,

Judy Huntress

ACKNOWLEDGMENTS

With a strong desire to honor caregivers, I embarked upon interviewing and talking with numerous people who had been caregivers or recipients of others' acts of kindness while faced with medical challenges. As I traveled the writer's path of gathering information for *Caregivers: Angels without Wings*, I met innumerable people who willingly shared their experiences and lessons they learned on their journeys. It has been an emotional trip completed as a labor of love. Along the way, I met wonderful people, some who became good friends even though we have never met in person.

I thank my family and friends who allowed me to talk incessantly about what I had learned from others, crying and laughing with me as I shared the compassionate and heart warming stories I heard along the way. They listened and gave feedback as I bounced ideas off them about the creation of *Caregivers: Angels without Wings*.

Special Tribute

An extra special tribute is given to the following people who assisted me in this labor of love.

Marv Crandall, my husband and mainstay, provided moral support and was exceptionally patient as I spent uncountable hours in our study writing when he would have preferred for us to be out enjoying retirement, a new stage in our lives. His encouragement never wavered. I am especially grateful for the hours and talents he contributed while editing the manuscript.

Judy Huntress, my sister, who surprised me the morning prior to submitting the manuscript to the publisher. She called and said, "Peg, I would like for you to include a page, which I am faxing, in your book. It is with deep gratitude that I include her loving and compassionate letter to caregiving readers, as the foreword to this book.

Jack and Katie Haley, my son and daughter, provided constant encouragement and contributed their talents during the creation of this book. Jack relieved my frustration with his solutions to technical computer problems I encountered along the way. Katie's creative talent came forth as she developed the design concept for the cover of *Caregivers: Angels without Wings*. I am grateful for their help, moral support, and love.

Sandra Lahr, friend, oncology nurse, and support group facilitator at the Nevada Cancer Center, made significant contributions to the *Relationships* chapter and provided guidance based on her professional experience. I sincerely appreciate her willingness to take time from her busy schedule to edit the manuscript and give words of encouragement.

Julie Neumeier, friend and neighbor, who willingly edited the manuscript and shared knowledge she gained from the book with a family member who had just become a caregiver. I thank Julie for her input and appreciate her passing on words of wisdom to a caregiver.

Story Contributors

I am forever grateful to the following people who were willing to share chapters of their lives, with the hope that their stories and advice will smooth the path for other caregivers. Patti Andersun, Darrell Bradley, Larry Carlson family, Jennifer Daniels, Jill DiLoretto, Kim Dwire, Sylvia Freeman, Bob and Judy Ginsberg, Karen Goodkind, Patti Gragg, Laura Gross, Greg Harris, Mona Jackson, Ginger Jacob, Ed Jensen, Ronnie Kaye, Barbara Lewis, Jacinta Lewis, Suzanne Lichtenberger, Mary McConnell, Patty Michael, Jan Nicholl, Carol Mooney, Debbie Reynolds, Marlee Rogow, Andy Rogers, Suzanne Rosa, Kathy Saxe, Earlene Taylor, and those who chose to remain anonymous.

Input From Many

Caregivers: Angels without Wings would not be complete without the extensive input from people I met along the way. Although they have not shared specific stories, their words of wisdom and encouragement for caregivers are woven into the fabric of this book.

Nevada Cancer Support Group

Sara Anderson, Mary and Sonny Bowman, Susan Rush, Jim and Cathy Clayton, Gene Goldman, Dorothy Hartsell, Diann Kukla, Mark Oatman, Connie and Perry Pearlstein, Keith and Mary Russell, Larry and Kelly Sheckler, Carmen and Vito Stolfa. In addition to those named above and to those who contributed stories, I extend my sincere gratitude to all members of our Monday night support group. It is impossible to list everyone who has become entwined within these pages through their shared thoughts and feelings about caregiving.

Avon Breast Cancer 3 Day

I am grateful for the enthusiasm and efforts of the Avon *3 Day* coaches who asked walkers if they would like to share their stories in this book. The walkers' response was incredible and the opportunity to interview these people would not have happened without the walker-coaches spreading the word.

All who are a Part of *Caregivers: Angels without Wings*

Even though not named there are a multitude of caregivers, people with medical problems, health care professionals, family members, friends, and acquaintances who have influenced the writing of *Caregivers: Angels without Wings*. Please know that you have a part within the pages of this book and a special place in my heart.

Introduction

"The repercussion of a person's serious disease ripples through the lives of many. A loved one may suffer with physical health issues but family and friends carry the burden with gentle hands and a heavy heart."

—An Anonymous Caregiver

Word spreads quickly when someone is diagnosed with a serious disease or disability. Friends, family, co-workers, and even acquaintances are affected. The initial news may leave you feeling emotional, stunned, and helpless because you don't know which way to turn. It is my hope that you will find this book valuable as an aid to smooth your caregiving journey.

Caregiving ranges from daily intervention with one who is ill to simply sending a "thinking of you" card. The extent of involvement of those in *Caregivers: Angels without Wings* range from primary to occasional to caregiving from a long distance.

As you read the portrayals of caregivers' experiences, you might find yourself smiling at their humor or perhaps even shedding compassionate tears as you relate to their journeys. Connecting with the people who shared their stories may give you needed emotional support that jumps from the page into your heart. Lessons learned along the way are included in the *Words of Wisdom* sections, as well as the handy checklists in the final chapter.

The purpose of this book is to honor caregivers, share their experiences, and provide moral support, encouragement, and practical tips for those who find themselves wearing a caregiver's hat. The specific disease is not the issue. It is the strength gained by caregivers who share and learn from one another ; it is the universal challenges, rewards, and day-to-day happenings that bring caregivers together.

Caregivers' Checklists

As I listened to caregivers, they often told me that, when a thought popped into their minds about what needed to be done or how they could brighten the day for their ailing friend, they wrote notes on scraps of paper. Post-it notes could be found throughout their homes and offices attached to refrigerator doors, bathroom mirrors, and computer screens. Many conveyed a need to organize and pinpoint specific suggestions that would be helpful for others as they made their way as a caregiver.

An answer to their request is the *Caregivers' Checklists* found in the final chapter of *Caregivers: Angels without Wings*. These handy lists are a compilation of caregivers' and patients' suggestions that supplement the *Words of Wisdom*. They include practical, universal suggestions for caregivers, regardless of the physical problem their friend or family member faces. The intent is to help caregivers and to provide suggestions for their support people in determining what they can do to share the care.

Epiphany—How this Book Came to Be

I was diagnosed with breast cancer three weeks prior to relocating from Maryland to Nevada. As we were flying cross-country to our new home, my husband, Marv, sat next to me working word puzzles. I enjoyed the quiet time, reflecting on the gifts of friendship, love, and support I had already been given when people heard about my diagnosis. I thought about my sister who had the same type of cancer three years earlier. We both had marveled at the outpouring of love and support we received from friends, family, and acquaintances.

Marv suddenly asked, "Peg, why don't you retire?"

"I don't think I'm ready," I said.

Whoops! I no more than finished that statement when I felt a flash that lit up my heart. I knew it was an epiphany in my life.

I said, "Marv, I've changed my mind. I will retire. I'm going to write a book about and for caregivers. I want to honor the wingless angels who give of themselves to friends and family who battle disease. I'll ask them to share their experiences, feelings, and advice. If they are willing, I'll share their stories with others who can benefit from what they have endured."

He expressed his full support of my new endeavor.

Wanting to Share

As I began interviewing caregivers, I found they were more than willing to talk about those chapters in their lives, anxious to tell of their difficulties as well as the sweet moments. They revealed lessons learned, emotional journeys, and described the lasting impressions the experience had on them personally. They were eager to pass on their stories and words of wisdom to other caregivers.

This book is my gift to present and future caregivers, and my way of honoring, paying tribute, to those who have already traveled that road.

Many stories are told just as they happened; others are anthologies based on a myriad of conversations with caregivers and patients. Some of the names are real; others have been changed for privacy reasons.

This is not a book on physical health care. Although not medically substantiated, all the stories and words of wisdom contain the essence of what it is to be a caregiver, whether on a full-time basis or one that is not quite so demanding.

A Note of Thanks

I extend my sincere appreciation to those who so willingly unfolded a piece of themselves so other caregivers might learn from their experiences and feel comfort in knowing they are not alone. Caregivers are truly *Angels without Wings*.

It is my hope that this book also fulfills, for others, the following wish of a woman who was her mother's caregiver.

"How I wish I had something like this to read during the three months I sat by my mother's bedside, gave her my love, and supported her through a very difficult time. It would have helped me to know I wasn't alone in such an ordeal, and I could have learned from those who have lived through similar challenges."

1

A Caregiver Is...

THE PRIMARY CAREGIVER

A Primary Caregiver's Balancing Act

"Lung cancer?" I asked in disbelief. "Doctor Sam, that's not possible. Dillon never smoked. How can he have lung cancer?"

My husband's oncologist replied, "We don't have all the answers. We've made great medical progress in treating cancer but I can't be certain as to what caused Dillon's disease."

We were shocked. We left Dr. Sam's office, still stunned. I felt like a robot, walking straight ahead through rows of cars in the parking lot, seemingly in a trance. Amazingly enough, we found our car. But before we opened the doors, we stood there looking at each other. We hugged for a long time, which helped ease us out of our state of bewilderment.

We weren't sure what to do next but knew we needed to do something. Stagnation, just waiting, was not our modus operandi. About an hour after we arrived home, we realized we had a burning need to learn all we could about this disease and potential treatments.

"Internet!" we both said at the same moment.

We were not surprised at our impromptu response. We began with the American Cancer Society website and continued with related links. We found a wealth of valuable information at our finger tips and needed to sort through the data to select relevant documentation. It was a quest that made us feel more upbeat because we knew Knowledge is Power.

The next morning, we each called our managers at work and told them about the recent developments. Of course, they understood we needed time off from work. I would be out at least two weeks to go with Dillon to what seemed like a zillion medical appointments for exams, procedures, and evaluations. The length of his medical leave remained to be seen.

What to tell our two children troubled us. They were only four and six years old. We wondered how much they could comprehend at their young ages. We decided not to tell them more than necessary, letting the depth of their questions be our guide.

The night before Dillon's surgery we knew it was time to talk with our son and daughter, Billy and Becky. Dillon tried to speak, but tears welled up in his eyes and he gulped as he tried to swallow the lump in his throat. He looked at me and shook his head. I knew he wanted me to take over. I explained that Daddy was going into the hospital for a few days and would have an operation. I told them that when he came home he probably would not feel like playing.

"Will his operation hurt?" Billy asked.

Becky wanted to know if he would have Sesame Street band-aids on his chest.

I answered their questions and we talked about a few changes they could expect in their routines. They suggested that they could help by being quiet while Daddy was resting. Dillon and I both smiled knowing that was not likely to happen.

Following Dillon's surgery and release from the hospital, I returned to work, resumed taking the kids to school and picking them up from their play groups at the end of the day, a routine that their dad had developed. I did all of the usual "Mom things" and made sure the kids and I continued our nightly ritual of reading books and singing together. I added the "Dad stuff" to my responsibilities so Dillon could rest.

Our neighbors, friends and family were wonderful. They called to check on Dillon's progress, brought meals to the house, gave us gift certificates for pizza to be delivered, and offered to take the children into their homes whenever needed or when we just wanted a little quiet time.

A few weeks after Dillon's surgery, I felt the outside world thought everything had returned to normal in our home. The frequent gifts of prepared meals decreased to almost zero. Rather than specific offers to help, our friends extended blanket invitations for us to let them know what they could do for us. I knew they were sincere in their willingness to help but I just couldn't bring myself to ask for assistance.

While at work, I thought my boss expected me to continue meeting the high standards I had set for myself throughout my career. That became difficult at times because my mind was often preoccupied with Dillon and all his diagnosis encompassed.

My job involved extensive travel. However, while Dillon was treated for cancer, I tried to avoid business trips. Then it became essential that I meet with clients on the east coast.

Dillon's mom and dad volunteered to take him to his chemo treatment and have him stay in their home while I was gone. I arranged for the children to spend a week with their grandparents, who lived out of town. Then I traveled cross country to a week filled with business obligations.

When I returned home, I was immersed in work and home responsibilities. I helped Dillon with his medications and continued with the never-ending household tasks and, of course, cared for our children. I couldn't leave Becky and Billy at home while their dad was feeling so poorly so I took them with me to run errands. That doubled the usual time required to complete those tasks.

After work, I helped Billy with his school work and Becky with her pre-school creative projects, made lunches for the next day, cleaned dinner dishes, helped the kids bathe, and put them into bed. I did all I could for Dillon but by the end of the day, when we sat down together, I was exhausted. I understood why he thought I was distant but I couldn't seem to do anything about it.

My stress level increased and my self-expectations laid heavy on my spirit. My physical health deteriorated. I was tired but didn't have time to rest. I was worn down and felt on edge, about to snap.

I needed to talk so I called my friend, Patty. She listened intently and then told me that her mother, Maya, had been her dad's primary caregiver while he was ill. She suggested I meet her mom and share my burden. Patty thought her mom was a wise woman and that she would be able to help me determine what I needed to do to alleviate some of my stress.

My Caregiver Coach

Maya and I met at a quaint Italian restaurant where they served delicious lasagna, one of my favorite entrees, at tables with white paper tablecloths and a bouquet of crayons that added color to the setting.

After the usual greetings, Maya said, "Elizabeth, the first lesson is the most difficult to learn. Once you accept it and realize it is a necessity, you will be better able to cope with your circumstances."

"What is it?" I asked.

"Recognize and accept change; change in your circumstances and in the way you manage your life. You need to reorganize and modify your priorities. You cannot be a primary caregiver and continue your life as though things were status quo. That's not realistic."

"But what can I do?" I asked.

She said, "SIMPLIFY! First, consider short-term and long-term commitments. Decide which of those you can set aside for the time being.

"Next, make a list of your everyday tasks and responsibilities. Organize your thoughts by creating an outline of your daily and weekly action items."

Maya selected a peacock blue crayon from the glass on our table. She handed it to me.

"Let's draft an outline to help you get started," she said.

As we talked about my responsibilities, I wrote:

I.   Dillon

    a. medications

    b. medical appointments

    c. time together

II.   Children

    a. attention

    b. meals

    c. physical needs

    d. driving them to and from school, day care, and their activities

III.   Work

    a. meetings

    b. travel

    c. conference calls

IV.   Household

    a. cleaning

    b. laundry

    c. meals

    d. errands

Maya said, "Looking at your outline, leads to the next step, one that is a significant challenge."

"What is that?" I asked.

She replied, "**Let go!** Look at the Caregiver Checklist I brought for you. Take the list home and give it some serious consideration. Highlight those tips you might use. Add your own ideas. Decide what you might have others handle for you. Indicate names of people you think would be willing to help with specific responsibilities.

"Next, **create a plan** to eliminate all but your most essential responsibilities. Then simply make a few phone calls and **ask for help**."

"But I don't want to ask for help," I said. "I don't want to be a burden. Besides that, I've always been independent and in control of my life."

Maya slid her coffee cup aside, placed her arms on the table and leaned forward.

"Listen closely," she said. "Your friends want to help. Their offers have decreased because you weren't telling them what you, Dillon or the kids need. You're trying to do it all yourself. Asking for assistance is not a sign of weakness. It is a gift to your friends and family—an opportunity for them to support you and Dillon during this difficult chapter of your lives. You need to **accept the fact that things have changed** and that you cannot meet all expectations, especially those you have placed on yourself.

"Which reminds me; can you delegate business trips to another employee or sit in on meetings via conference call?"

"I'll think about that, Maya," I answered.

She reached across the table and touched my hand.

She said, "There is one more thing I want you to know. As you travel through this epic in your journey of life, you will become more aware of your intuition, your spirit, those internal messages—whatever you may call that voice within. Listen closely. Guidance is right there. You just need to be open to receiving it."

Maya threw out some real challenges, but I knew I would heed her advice.

We paid for lunch and stood to say goodbye.

I said, "Many, many thanks, Maya. You've helped me alter my perspective of what is and isn't necessarily my sole responsibility. I'll get organized and find ways to simplify my daily life. I will ask for—and graciously accept—the willingness of friends to support my family."

"Just" A Caregiver

It was George's first time to attend the cancer support group with his wife, Marge.

He introduced himself by saying, "I'm just a caregiver."

We were all dumbfounded.

"JUST? JUST?" we asked in unison, as though we were a chorus in a live the-atrical production.

But that was no performance. It was real life, involving apprehension and fear for members of the group.

"George, let me ask you a question. What do you do to help your wife?" asked one of our caregivers.

He replied, "Well, Marge is often nauseous following her chemo treatments so I prepare food that doesn't make her feel sick. For instance, simply a few sniffs of a tomato-base sauce sends her stomach into a volcanic reaction. So I've learned to avoid tomatoes and cook healthy meals that she can enjoy."

George was talking but he seemed reticent and a little embarrassed about being in the spotlight. But that didn't stop any of us. "Just" was not in our vocab-ulary and we would not relent until he understood the critical role he was playing as his wife's caregiver while she was trying to defeat disease.

"What else do you do?" asked one our cancer patients.

"I keep the house clean," he said. He smiled at Marge and continued, "Until she got sick, I didn't realize the time and effort she put into maintaining our home in tip-top condition."

We all laughed.

Our group facilitator said, "Tell us other things you are doing to help Marge."

"I give her medications. I do the grocery shopping. I run all the errands," George answered.

Joe, another care-giving husband was in our circle that night.

He asked, "George do you go to medical appointments with Marge? Do you handle insurance problems?"

"Yes, I sure do," George replied. I'm with her at every doctor's appointment and sit with her while she receives chemotherapy. And insurance? I'm amazed at the quagmire of paper work and phone calls. There seems to be a never-ending need to solve insurance related problems."

"I bet you ask questions and do research on the internet about her condition, right?" Joe asked.

George answered, "Actually, I do all of those things. I remember finding some information about her particular type of cancer on a health-related website. I was unclear as to how it fit Marge's case so I took a printed copy to her oncologist. He explained everything to both of us. We were relieved to learn it was not the can of worms we thought we had opened."

Joe spoke up again and asked, "George, I'm asking you to understand what an important advocate you are for Marge at this time in her life. You are her main caregiver."

George nodded but did not seem fully convinced.

Our facilitator turned toward George's wife and said, "Now, let me ask you, Marge. How is he when it comes to emotional support?"

"Incredible," she replied. "I honestly don't think I could handle this without George's support. He listens. He lets me cry. He encourages me. And I treasure the times we simply sit together. I feel warm and safe when he puts his arm around me or holds my hand, not saying a word but simply being in the moment."

We broke into a spontaneous round of applause.

Marge continued, "I am in a critical period of my life and George is there to shore me up."

"Well, Mr.'Just' a Caregiver," another member said, "any new thoughts about your primary caregiver role in Marge's life?"

George paused. We could almost see thoughts flying through his mind. He looked at Marge and squeezed her hand. He looked around the circle. We were quiet but could feel something happen as his eyes met ours.

He spoke. We listened.

George said, "Now I understand the significance of my taking care of my wife. I'll stop minimizing the value of what I do for her. Thanks to all of you for opening my eyes. And one more thing—if I can help any of you, 'just' let me know."

We laughed again. That evening, every one of us left the meeting feeling uplifted. We knew we helped George understand the value of primary caregivers in the lives of those needing assistance while they confront a disease. He gained insight into why we honored him and every person who is a caregiver.

George seemed to realize what a positive impact he had on Marge's battle against cancer. He knew his efforts and love made a difference in how his wife felt. His tasks were seemingly endless and consumed most of his time and energy, but he would do all in his power to be her pillar of strength, her primary caregiver.

Words of Wisdom
Key Advice For All Primary Caregivers

You must take care of yourself in order to have the strength to support your special person who has been stricken with disease or disability. No doubt, you will want to focus all of your energies on your loved one. However, if you are worn out, feel fatigued, or drained emotionally, you will not have the energy to carry out your own commitment to give your best to your patient.

It is essential that you know "full-time" does not mean twenty-four hours a day with no time for your own rest, exercise, healthy eating, or mental and spiritual rejuvenation. Those who have been in that role, insist that you schedule a break for a few minutes each day, and time away from that environment at least twice a week. If necessary, ask a friend to sit in for you while you take a walk, ride your bicycle, play a round of golf, go to lunch with a friend, read a book, meditate, write in your journal, sit quietly and hold your cat, sip a cup of tea while inhaling nature's beauty, or simply just "be." Do something—or nothing at all—that leaves you feeling refreshed.

Flight attendants announce, "If the oxygen mask falls during flight, secure yours before helping someone traveling with you." Wise words. If you can't breathe, how can you care for the one with you? Obviously, the same applies to your care-giving circumstances. So take a deep breath of fresh air before diving back into your support role.

For additional tips, reference the chapter, *Attention Caregivers: How to Care for Yourself.*

She Learned to Recognize Her Own Time and Energy Limitations

- Accept change. At first, you may find it difficult to adjust; you may not recognize, or you may even deny the reality of the situation. However, it is essential to become aware of the fact that your usual routines need to be altered while you are in the role of a primary caregiver.

- Simplify. Outline your normal responsibilities. Decide what you must do yourself. Determine those tasks you can ask someone else to assume.

- Delegate. Know that your friends want to help. Give them the opportunity to support you and your loved one.

- Accept their help. Make it easier for them by letting them know exactly what they can do.

He Learned the Value of His Actions as a Primary Caregiver

- Know that you make a difference. Giving your time, energy, and support is a gift for the person who is sick.

- Do not minimize the value of your efforts. Realize how significant your support is for your loved one's physical and mental comfort.

- Feeling your efforts are insignificant is <u>not</u> allowed. Save humility for some other situation. Give yourself permission to accept gratitude and appreciation from your "patient" and others who care about that person.

- Join a support group of people who share similar experiences as caregivers. They will provide you with knowledge and, perhaps most importantly, strength and comfort.

OCCASIONAL CAREGIVERS

In the previous story, George was a primary caregiver. He soon found that caring for someone seriously ill or battling a disease often extends beyond the capabilities and energies of one human being.

Occasional caregivers are very special people who lend valuable assistance to primary caregivers and their loved ones who are struggling with disease. The time they give and their acts of kindness vary widely. They may prepare meals for the family, run errands, schedule appointments, care for the children, or sit with their friend so the primary caregiver can take a break; perhaps they might simply send a card or call now and then to say "I'm thinking of you."

Alice worked with Susan, whose sister had been diagnosed with multiple sclerosis. Alice assumed Susan's job responsibilities any time Susan needed to leave the office to take her sister to medical appointments. Ed drove his friend, Joe, to radiation treatments. Mary called Louise often to see how she was recovering from a stroke. For months, while Judy was receiving chemotherapy, her neighbors brought meals to her family. Co-workers and friends sent Mark cards, balloons, plants, books, and videos to brighten his days while he spent many weeks recovering from serious injuries he incurred in an auto accident. Joanne sat with Lou's wife while he took a break from his intense care-giving situation.

The number and types of acts of kindness provided by occasional caregivers is inexhaustible. Their part in caring for someone varies in time and type of involvement. The "once in a while caregivers" are extremely important for patients, primary caregivers, and their families. From the smallest gesture to assuming significant responsibilities are of great importance to the people dealing with disease or disability. Occasional caregivers discover that there is nothing quite like the feeling of satisfaction and joy of helping someone in need. You will find it rewarding.

Mel's friend was diagnosed with prostate cancer. The treatment left his friend weak and insecure about driving. Mel jumped right in and acted as his friend's chauffeur, not just for medical appointments, but also to take him anywhere else he needed or wanted to be.

A friend asked Mel, "Why do you do all of these things?"

He said, "Being there for others in need is just a part of my life. It's what I do."

People like Mel are proactive. They seek answers to the question, "What can I do to ease their stress?"

They simply take the initiative to make things happen.

They make a phone call and ask, "What can I do to help?" or say, "I'll pick up Carrie and Joey after school today; I'll be there about five o'clock with your dinner; or I'm going to the grocery store, anything you need?"

Good Intentions but Not the Foggiest Idea of What to Do

Do you want to help someone who is sick but do not know what to do or even where to begin? The *Caregivers' Checklists* in the final chapter of this book relays numerous ideas and suggestions for the varying roles of caregivers. People involved in these situations have emphasized the importance of each gesture and act of kindness that eases the difficulties of day-to-day life, for anyone involved with health battles.

Ask what you can do. Add your own ideas to the checklist. Keep the tips handy as a reminder of specific ways you can help as an occasional caregiver. Remember—giving care occasionally is a great gift!

CAREGIVER AND PATIENT—CONCURRENTLY

Going It Alone

I was the one with cancer. I had to step out of myself and be my own caregiver. I had to wake myself up and do for me. I learned the buck stops here. I became incredibly brave. I had some type of maternal instinct to take care of myself. I had to call the doctor, schedule mammograms, handle insurance problems, and convince administrators that even though I was self-insured, there was a cache of money for this purpose.

Strength! I was so strong for my inner child. I knew I had to save this person diagnosed with breast cancer. Nothing to do but to do it. I marched from the oncologist to the radiologist. I was on a mission.

Then the radiation diminished my physical health. I was drained emotionally. I realized that it was preposterous to do all of this alone. I could no longer go home and be silent. I had a driving need to talk.

I told my oncologist about my state of mind. He gave me the name of the facilitator of a support group at a local cancer center. I attended the meetings where people encouraged me to talk about my situation. They listened. They shared their knowledge and supported me with compassion. They laughed at my jokes and antics. They were the reason I made it through a terribly difficult ordeal.

I am grateful for the support they gave me to meet the challenges of battling disease on my own, facing fears, emotional trauma, and finding courage I did not know I had. With their encouragement, I succeeded as my own primary caregiver.

I Was My Only Caregiver—So I Thought

This is the story of a man who was alone, cynical, and suffering with multiple myeloma. During his ordeal, he moved from a place of complete negativity to a fully positive approach to life. His metamorphosis shone through his smile as he touched the lives of other cancer patients and their caregivers.

Although I had experienced sporadic back pain for three years, I was completely taken by surprise the day I felt spasms so intense that I could not stand. I fell to the floor in agony. I was alone. I needed help. The pain finally subsided enough that I could drag myself across my living room floor to the telephone. I called a friend from work.

He came to my apartment, took one look at me, and dialed 911. The ambulance arrived within minutes. The paramedics propped up my body with theirs as I made a strong effort to walk to the ambulance. At the hospital, they placed me on a gurney and wheeled me into the emergency room, where a quick diagnosis was made.

The ER physician said, "Back pain. I can't feel anything out of place. I'll prescribe some pain medication to be taken every four hours so you can return to work."

I thought, "I have no choice but to work. If I don't, I can't pay the rent or my bills."

I did go to work but the medication had me feeling and acting like a space cadet.

During the evenings at home, loneliness set in big time! I've lived alone most of my adult life but I have never felt such a strong need for another person's companionship and help as I did one week later when the pain recurred. I felt like crying but I could not let myself do that. I believed I had to be stoic, strong, and unflinching to get myself through this.

I remember thinking, "If only I had someone to talk with, someone to listen, and to explain to me what is happening to my body."

The pain was intense. I dialed 911. Once again, the paramedics wheeled me into the hospital on a gurney. Three emergency room doctors ran tests and could find no source of the problem. When they told me to stand, I could not, so two orderlies sat me up in bed. The awful scream that involuntarily came from my body did get their attention. Dr. Samson finally ordered several pulmonary tests because my breathing was abnormal. My blood cell counts were low. My back continued to give me excruciating pain.

After three weeks of tests, a new doctor approached my bed. I could not read his nametag but I could see the word embroidered on his white coat. "Oncologist."

"This is it" I thought, "I have cancer."

"Donald," he said, "you have multiple myeloma, a cancer that attacks plasma cells. When the cells grow out of control, they can form tumors, typically in the soft middle parts of bone marrow. I'm prescribing chemotherapy."

The doctor called in a medical social worker, who helped me arrange for treatment. Then I was released from the hospital. I went home to my seemingly empty apartment. For a few days, the only thing I could do was focus on getting rid of the pain and learning to walk again. All that accompanied with a deep sense of loneliness.

About a week later, I began calling my co-workers, who I thought were friends. One guy was willing to write checks to pay my bills. I signed them. He took the envelopes to the mail box. Other so-called friends had nothing to say and did not want to come to visit. I was amazed to find my "friends" were not there in time of need. I felt like someone who had the plague; forlorn, abandoned and terribly lonely.

Every day I asked myself, "Who can I really trust? Is anyone out there who can help?"

I could think of no one other than myself. I was in a new town and had met very few people. With rare exception, those I did know avoided me once they knew I had cancer. I realized I was alone.

I had to be my own caregiver. I handled things well emotionally and I was resolute. Will power had taken me through tough times before and I knew I could do it again. With that determination in my hip pocket, I pursued my medical treatments.

During my first visit to the cancer center where I received chemotherapy, I met an oncology nurse, Nancy, who turned out to be an angel in disguise. She was willing to help in any way possible. Her knowledge was invaluable and her compassion gave me strength. Facing financial instability, she suggested I contact Medicare for disability assistance. Then she directed me to a number of sources that provided financial assistance and other support services for patients, including cancer organizations, medical groups and pharmaceutical companies.

Meanwhile, Nancy encouraged me to attend the Monday night support group meetings for cancer patients and their caregivers. I was hesitant at first. I was not at a trusting point in my life and did not know how I could share my problems with complete strangers.

I thought, "Everyone else has turned away from me; why would these people be any different?"

But, mostly for Nancy, I attended one of the meetings. When I discovered I was the only one with myeloma, I did not think I could gain anything from the group. But the next Monday rolled around and I decided to attend again. After all, at least I could be with people. Perhaps I would be able to socialize with them a bit.

After the first few minutes of that second meeting, I began to talk about my situation. Any doubts I had about people in that support group, went up in smoke. They became like family. It was the only place I felt I could talk about cancer without offending someone. Not only could I talk—they listened! People living with cancer and their caregivers provided me with incredible support. I began to believe I was not in this alone.

One of the men and I became good friends and I began to go out socially with him and his buddies. My world was looking brighter. Through that group of caring people I learned a great deal about cancer and even more about friendship and compassion.

A member of our Monday night group actually gave me a computer. What a fantastic tool. It threw open doors for me. I learned to search the internet. I read everything I could find about my disease. One path led to another. Opportunities for assistance, medically and financially, appeared on the screen. I became the group expert on finding relevant information and was able to share that knowledge. I began to gain self-confidence.

Then one Monday night, a guest speaker addressed our group as part of the *I Can Cope* program sponsored by the American Cancer Society.

"Listen closely to what she is saying," I thought. "I feel like she is touching the depths of my inner self. I want to talk to her privately after the presentation."

That was the beginning of a relationship with another angel. Melinda talked about creating your own reality and how to develop new ways of thinking; to move from negative expectations and be ready to accept positive reactions from others. That's exactly what I needed—and wanted—to do.

I met with her. She explained her counseling services and the fee structure. Payment was impossible for me. I had no source of funds to pay for counseling. But—not to worry. Melinda said she could see my strong need to change my perspective of life. She was willing to work with me at no charge.

I was dying of multiple myeloma. I felt abandoned by family and friends, except for my Monday night support group. Melinda and I talked a great deal about my childhood and how I was allowing those difficult times to let me believe I deserved to suffer with cancer.

I discovered that I was setting myself up for rejection. When I met someone new, I initiated conversation by immediately bringing up the topic of my disease. I told everyone about my severe back pain and what it was like to be poked with needles, feeling like a giant pin cushion. I finally realized that they must have felt they were being prodded with surgical instruments and chose to leave the scene of an operating room.

Melinda helped me to discard my blinders that were causing tunnel vision. It took a while, but once I was able to alter my own perspective of life, my whole world opened up. *I learned that a person creates his or her own reality every day. By choice, we react positively or negatively to people and circumstances.* I needed to deal with my feelings and things other than cancer that were happening in my life. When I felt off-balance I looked at what was bothering me and dealt with that. I learned that a spiritual flow is always present; I just needed to open myself to the universe and allow the spirit to reignite within me.

During the time I worked with and learned from Melinda, I inherited a small (huge in my situation) amount of money. I planned to buy a car and pay bills but Melinda encouraged me to first travel to California to receive a stem cell transplant.

I agreed and began another round of contacting health care professionals and making arrangements for travel. I needed financial assistance and was able to find it through a cancer organization.

I was nervous the day I drove five hours to the facility. It was the first time I had actually driven by myself to a large city and navigated my way around on major freeways. I found the hospital, the hotel, and even allowed myself to walk on the beach. That in itself was comforting.

My medical team was excellent. They too cared for me with compassion. The stem cell transplant was successful and within a couple of days I drove back home. Six months later, I returned for a follow-up exam. I was elated with the reception I received from the entire medical team. The doctor at the clinic talked to me about living with a chronic illness, <u>not</u> looking at cancer as a disease that was taking my life.

My attitude changed. My life was wonderful, I laughed a lot, I met new people with more confidence, and I looked forward to every day. I realized how I created my own reality.

I was my only caregiver when this epic began. Now I know I am my strongest support person but not the only one.

The Monday night support group admired Donald's perseverance, resourcefulness, his self-taught knowledge, and—most of all—his bright, cheerful attitude. He became a hero and mentor for many, especially those who are diseased and are their own primary caregiver.

A Wake Up Call

I noticed people in the mall doing a double take, another glance over their shoulder to see if their eyes were playing tricks on them. I was certain they were wondering why a bald-headed woman would be entering a beauty salon. That woman with no hair was me, a cancer patient and a hair stylist. I was going to work.

Tissue very close to my heart carried inflammatory cancer. My physicians told me they were amazed that I was still walking. I was the only person they knew who was living with that threatening condition.

The critical point is, I was alive—walking, working, and loving my family and friends. I resolved to have a positive attitude, to get out of bed each morning, and to be active. I had a wake-up call and heeded the message.

Patients made a special effort to come to our salon to talk with me.

I told them, "If I start my day feeling negative, that's what I will receive—negativity. But I have the power to change what will happen to me. I take an affirmative stance; I seek positive energy and return the same to those around me."

Disease took me to many different levels of questioning—and answering—but I guess I did not really consider myself a caregiver for other cancer victims until it was called to my attention that I was doing more than battling my own disease; I was providing support for other women affected by cancer. I have always cared deeply about people but cancer patients assumed a special place in my heart.

I've been amazed at how many women have come to me because someone told them, "Deanna will make you feel better."

A man brought his wife into the shop for a haircut. He asked for me by name. I asked why they (only to learn it was he, not they) specifically requested my services.

He said, "A friend told me you could help."

His wife had been lying in bed for four weeks. The skin under her eyes had already turned a dark grey, almost black, and she was terribly thin because she refused to eat. Her hair was tangled into a mat like a rat's nest. I had no choice but to cut her hair so short that you could see the skin on her head.

Then I began my verbal assault.

I said, "You are already dead. Look at you. You are terrorizing your entire family and preying on their pity. Are you craving so much attention that you have gone to such extremes? You had a biopsy and four rounds of chemo. You've been behaving as though your life is over. Wake up! You are still here and you are so fortunate to have a family who loves and supports you."

Her facial muscles tightened, she gritted her teeth, and she glared at me through her squinted eyes. I knew she was furious.

Challenging me, she said, "I don't believe you went back to work just four weeks after surgery, especially having had lymph nodes removed. I do not believe that was possible."

I said, "I could not—and would not—just lie in bed. I forced myself to get up, dress, and go to work. The first few weeks I folded towels rather than styling hair but that helped me regain strength in my arm that was weakened by the surgical procedure that removed lymph nodes. Perhaps even greater than physical recovery was the joy I felt in my heart."

She left the salon, visibly upset.

I thought, "Aha! I've achieved my goal. Anger is a motivator and I've set a fire under her."

A week later, her husband stopped by to see me.

He said, "We all want to thank you for rekindling my wife's desire to live. She's out of bed, even taking morning walks, and eating again. She smiles, laughs and talks with all of us. You've given her the drive to move forward and you've given me my wife, whom I thought I had lost."

I was ecstatic that she was rebounding and grateful that I was able to help.

Another lady came to see me. She had brain cancer and her oncologist had told her the prognosis was one year to live.

With that in mind she said, "A friend told me about your positive approach to life. But knowing I have just one year left, how can you make me positive?"

I said, "I don't expect you to be positive all the time. But I would like to see you share your strength with others. You came here today. That took affirmative steps on your part."

We talked for an hour. We joked and laughed about my being bald and envious of her hair. She told me details about her cancer and her feelings concerning the doctors' pronouncement that she had only one year left on this planet.

I said, "I believe no one can be certain of when any person will die. Life may last another fifty years or could be snuffed out in a moment. You are alive today and express more enthusiasm than many people on the street. You appreciate life. I share that attitude with you. I am happy that I can stand in a line at the grocery store, sit in traffic, see a child smile…each day you and I have is one of joy."

"Okay Deanna. I hear you," she said.

A few weeks later, she returned to the salon.

She said, "Since our conversation, I found myself walking down the street noticing people with drooped heads or wearing frowns on their faces. I want to walk right up and say, 'Good grief. Do you know what you're missing? Smile. Only you can change your attitude.'"

I gave her a big hug. I loved being around her because she had such an uplifting attitude, in spite of her prognosis. We agreed to have a nutritious lunch together the following week.

I know that positive energy surrounds all of us. One simply needs to open their eyes, mind, and heart to let the force I call "positivity" fill their very being.

The Energizer Bunny

This is the story of a woman who cared for her husband, a stroke victim, while she battled ovarian cancer.

Early on a Tuesday evening, Dave, my husband, had difficulty speaking and felt some weakness in his right hand. Over the next several hours, the symptoms worsened. By the next morning, his entire right side was affected. I knew pitifully little about stroke and found I was scared to death.

Dave was hospitalized in the intensive care unit all night. After he was stabilized, I went home to clean up and change clothes. I spent about ten minutes in the shower crying. Then I got my act together.

After I returned to the hospital, Dave's folks left and drove the fifty miles to their home. Carl, our son, stayed for a while and then went home to get some sleep. I spent most of the night thinking about what I needed to do but reached very few conclusions. Stroke symptoms are too visible to deny and I was terribly scared and confused.

Although I tended to be very practical and managed my display of emotions, I certainly felt them. Dave had always told me I just didn't express my feelings enough.

But I often told him, "If I don't display great elation and go 'nutso' with excitement, that doesn't mean I'm not happy and feeling joyous about things."

Conversely, when bad things happened, I didn't suffer the depths of depression. I guess I always felt that was a good trade-off.

However, in this situation, I wanted to hold Dave and show him my love. We hugged a lot for the first few hours until he was not aware of what was going on around him. That syndrome lasted for several days. I did take walks and cried, but I tried not to let the tears flow when I was around *Dave*.

I was not known to be the quiet type. I talked to anyone who was willing to share their knowledge about strokes, rehabilitation, and treatment. I also talked with our family about what I needed to consider in preparing for Dave's homecoming. The doctors had told me the affects of the stroke were long term. Dave was unable to speak. He could not move any part of the right side of his body and could not swallow. For the time being, there was no decision that had to be made. It was simply that he needed to be in a rehabilitation hospital. He stayed two and a half months.

The best thing I did was to learn all I could about rehab methods. I researched various sources of information, talked with physical therapists, medical social workers, psychologists, and doctors.

I returned to work almost immediately after Dave's stroke. I went to the hospital every evening and stayed long hours on weekends. That is when my co-workers began to kid me about being the Energizer Bunny.

Carl decided not to return to an out-of-state college.

He said, "Mom, I can't leave you alone to cope with this and, besides, since I've been through almost every kind of physical rehab there is for my athletic injuries, I think I can help Dad."

Carl was a great support for me and a super caregiver for his father.

Emotions Surfaced

I was surprised to discover the extent of my emotions. I felt fear, anger, grief, guilt, confusion, doubt, and resentment. Denial really was not possible. Unlike some diseases, stroke symptoms hit you right in the face. My fear, confusion, and doubt, centered mainly on my how I could cope with everything. I grieved for Dave because I felt he did not deserve this. Anger and resentment came about because I had nagged him about smoking and losing some weight but he hadn't done anything to improve his health.

However, the ability to cope with the changes in our lives sort of took care of itself. I just did what I needed to do for Dave. I had lots of support from my son and Dave's folks.

I guess I never did get over the grief. Dave is a special kind of person who attracts people like a magnet, especially young people. In fact, even with his limited physical movement men, women and children were drawn to him. I knew it would be much more fun for all of us if he could speak and be more active. But I needed to accept reality; his condition was not likely to improve.

I gave up the anger and resentment early on after I asked myself, "What's the use of dwelling on the negative?"

I let it go. I believed more in action than in anger.

Financial Concerns

My worst worry was about our financial future. I couldn't discuss the state of affairs with Dave, so I turned to his parents and Carl. I spent quite a bit of time working on a budget and devising methods to save money however possible. As things turned out, I made enough to get along comfortably, which was a very pleasant surprised.

Daily Routines

We eased into our new daily routines, although it wasn't always easy. For instance, Dave needed specific daily exercise. He always worked on rehabilitation better with someone else than he did with me. I was really hurt when he would not work with me. Then the rehab psychologist explained that this was very, very common.

She said, "You're his wife, not his therapist."

His—and my—greatest frustration was his inability to talk. When he became angry, he swore. I do give him credit for learning to control those outbursts to "Gol darn!" I was amazed that he could say certain words but not converse. That's one of the side effects of a stroke.

A couple of times, out of frustration, my anger flared up. I tried so hard to help Dave rehabilitate and he just did not want to do his share of the work.

He gained fifty pounds. I said, "Dave, you will kill yourself if you don't do something about your weight. You will need to go to a nursing home if you cannot walk enough to maintain muscle tone in your right leg. I can't take care of you if you are unable to walk."

He put forth more effort after that encounter.

Then I Became the Patient

Two years after Dave's stroke, I was diagnosed with ovarian cancer. I began another quest for knowledge. By that time, I had medical research experience. I knew how to approach, discover, and sort through medical documentation. I had learned the types of questions to ask health care professionals. On the day my cancer was confirmed, my oncologist introduced me to the subject of ovarian cancer. Most of my information came from my oncologist, clinical nurses, and the *American Cancer Society*. I verified facts and advice on the internet. I called friends, who told me about women they knew who had ovarian cancer. I made many new friends through this networking process and learned a great deal about how to cope.

I recommend anyone, patient or caregiver, involved with a disease to become educated about the disease, treatment, and related changes in behavior. Ask questions! Ask questions! Ask questions!

Every time I met with my oncologist I had a written list of questions. He was always willing to talk. I learned about what was happening to my body and how to try to handle the pain, the effects of chemotherapy, and what foods were most suited for me.

My Caregivers

I had incredible support. Family members and friends were wonderful. Carl was the greatest. Dave, although limited in what he could do, wanted to support me in every way possible. He helped around the house and even found a way to prop himself against the kitchen counter so he could empty the dishwasher. He managed to fold laundry. I was amazed at how he developed his own system to tackle tasks such as folding king-sized sheets while sitting in a wheel chair. I was highly impressed by what he learned to do, simply out of sheer will power.

Our neighbors were extraordinary! The kids in the neighborhood mowed the lawn and they would not accept pay. Their mom wanted them to learn what it is to be part of a community. Another family held many celebrations throughout the year. During each of their events, they brought food to us.

Dave loved to be outside on his scooter. He could get around and socialize, even though he could not talk. One Saturday morning, an old friend saw him driving through the neighborhood. She followed him home and visited with us for a while. The next day her husband came over and installed a lift in the trunk of our car so I could take Dave's scooter with us when we went out. What a difference that made! We were able to go places more often. Our friends' gift continued to lift our spirits, as well as his scooter.

I continued to work for six years after my diagnosis. My friends from work were thoughtful and supportive while I received chemotherapy and continued to care for Dave. They marveled at how I handled my own treatment, cared for Dave, continued to perform my job, being there for the students and co-workers in the Student Union. My nickname, "Energizer Bunny," spread throughout the faculty and student body at the university.

I loved my job but my health finally dictated that I needed to retire. A very large group of friends—students, staff, administrators, and faculty, attended my retirement party. The staff found one person whom I hadn't seen for fifteen years. She attended my party. I received cards and flowers sent from all over the country. I cannot explain how extraordinary my work and the people were for me.

Once medically retired, I continued to hear from those I had known while working as office manager in the Student Union. Their outpouring of support was like a bright beam coming from a lighthouse in the midst of darkness.

I began to feel isolated. I missed being involved with people at work. However, I found e-mail to be an especially wonderful means of communicating while living within my circumstances. I received daily messages from my friends. I even received e-mails from as far away as Pakistan, from a former student who heard I was not doing well and contacted me immediately.

I extend my deepest gratitude to all who shored me up during those eight trying years. I will always treasure their love and thoughtfulness.

Connie passed away after six years of a valiant fight against ovarian cancer. The Energizer Bunny is sorely missed. Dave continues to live at home with the help of a daily caregiver and with the amazing care and concern of family and very special neighbors.

Words of Wisdom
Patient and Caregiver Concurrently

It has been said often, "I think it must be more difficult to be a caregiver than to be the patient."

Most caregivers flatly refute that statement. There is no right or wrong answer in this debate. However, if you need to integrate being a caregiver and a patient at the same time, the challenges are immense.

Men and women who traveled the dual pathway shared the following advice. Some were patients, alone, while being their own caregiver; others wrestled with their own disease while caring for someone else who was sick or incapacitated. Their dual perspectives provide insight on how to handle such a difficult journey.

They suggest that you may be resentful about carrying such a heavy weight. At the same time, you probably "clam up" and bear heavy-duty emotions within yourself. That creates stress, which can lead to worsening your health. The bottom line is to open up!

- Reach out for support. Talk to friends, a counselor, health care social workers, nurses, support groups; tell someone how you are feeling.

- Write letters to an understanding friend.

- Take pen in hand and write your feelings and thoughts in your personal journal.

- Ask your oncology health professionals for sources of information.

- Think "outside the box." Pursue all leads for assistance.

- Do something for yourself that is not disease-related. Go to a movie, a museum, a park. Walk on the beach.

- Give some thought to Donald's lesson: "I learned that a person creates his or her own reality every day. By choice, we react positively or negatively to people and circumstances."

ACROSS THE MILES

The Plus Side of Long Distance Caregiving

My work required frequent travel and my conscience bothered me because I could not spend more time with my best friend while she battled a life-threatening disease. As her condition worsened, I felt very guilty about not being able to be at her bedside.

I talked with my therapist about my feelings. She explained that many seriously ill patients find their favorite relationships to be with those who stay in touch by phone. There is sound reasoning behind that point. When people visit a very sick person face to face, they often treat him or her as fragile beings that need to be handled with kid gloves. That behavior makes the one who is ill feel they have lost their self-identity and are nothing more than a medical problem.

However, when telephone calls replace in-person visits, normal conversations take place because the caregiver does not see her friend's deteriorating physical appearance. That is a plus. It prevents tension that the caregiver might otherwise experience.

In retrospect, I must admit that when I was out of town I did not treat June differently when we talked on the phone; however, when I saw her in pain and withering away, I was very uncomfortable.

Seeing someone looking gaunt and grim, makes it difficult to sit down and say, "Wow. What a day I've had. Let me tell you…"

Even though I tried to be my usual self, it was tough, and I found myself wearing those soft kid gloves.

I have thought a lot about our long-distance relationship and realized there were some other advantages to being apart. If I had been with her, she would have tried to stay awake and talk, even when she needed to rest. Another plus for both of us was the fun we had when I called. We would just chat for a few minutes and then I surprised her by playing one of her favorite songs or having a mutual friend say hello.

Geographic separation from a loved one who is suffering with pain may be excruciating for caregivers but staying in touch via phone, just hearing that person's voice, brings relief.

As the AT&T slogan puts it, "Reach out and touch someone." It feels good. It is good.

A Continent Apart Is Difficult For Mom

I live in the northeast where the land is touched by the waves of the Atlantic Ocean. I've often felt solace by merely listening to the sound of the waves rushing in and watching the beauty of the white foamy surf. As the waves waned and were pulled back out to sea, I knew they would return. I walked on the beach and inhaled the wonder of it all, feeling comfort and peace.

But when my daughter, Susan, was diagnosed with breast cancer, I was not ready to handle the ongoing rising and waning of waves of emotions that recurred frequently. It was very difficult to be almost 3,000 miles away from her while she was undergoing a number of surgeries and chemotherapy. The fact that she was thirty years old and married did not make it any easier. Your child is your child, regardless of age or marital status.

We received a great deal of support from Charles, Susan's husband. Just knowing he was with her relieved a lot of anxiety that my husband, Bruce, and I felt about not being able to be by her side. He supported Susan emotionally and cared for her in all ways possible.

Susan discovered a lump in her breast and immediately went to her primary care physician, who referred her to an oncologist. Calcifications run in the family so we were not overly concerned. My sister had them. I've had them. I was certain the findings would be the same for Susan.

The oncologist proposed doing a biopsy but Susan elected to have a lumpectomy. She wanted to be certain about what was happening in her body. I think she had a strong feeling that it was cancer and I believe the oncologist felt the same.

When the lumpectomy revealed the tumors were malignant, we were shocked into accepting that her young age did not make her immune to this disease. More decisions needed to be made concerning her next step and ongoing treatment. She and Charles made sound decisions while my husband, Bruce and I tried not to express our opinions. She had brain scans, bone scans, mammograms and surgery after surgery. Even after she had gone through chemotherapy, the radiologist discovered another lump and scheduled yet another surgical procedure. Fortunately, that time they discovered a benign cyst. However, with the way things had been going, waiting a week to hear the results was about as easy as sailing a boat in a hurricane.

I was working at home one Thursday afternoon. The phone rang. Bad news always seemed to come on Thursdays. I hurried to pick up the receiver.

I heard Susan say, "Hi Mom. I just had a follow-up appointment with my doctor. He discovered more cancer in my breast. I need a mastectomy."

I felt like I was thrown overboard. I was not prepared for the news even though I probably should have been. After all, the surgeon removed ten lymph nodes when he performed the lumpectomy. I guess nothing could ready me for the ongoing challenges Susan faced. That was the only time I lost control while talking with my daughter. Tears streamed down my face and she could hear me sob.

She asked "Are you alright Mom?"

"Not really," I answered. "Is it alright if we call when your father returns from work?"

She said, "Of course Mom. I'll talk to you later."

I pondered how I could tell Bruce about the latest development. It had been so difficult for him to receive news second hand and this was going to be a real blow. About that time, he walked in the door.

After our usual greetings, I took a deep breath and said, "Bruce—Susan called and we need to call her back."

I told him, briefly, about the findings and the need for a mastectomy. He was stunned and speechless. We dialed the phone. Susan gave us the details.

After that phone conversation, Bruce did something he had never done before. He yelled at me. I think he was so devastated about the news that his pain and anger erupted. I had heard that people under stress, lash out at those with whom they are closest. That was the only time he reacted in that manner. Actually, throughout this entire ordeal we felt exceptionally close to one another.

Susan was strong and, when necessary, took aggressive steps regarding her medical care. For instance, at one point she tried to make an appointment for a mammogram.

"Ten days before we have an opening," she was told.

That was not acceptable! She needed one now! She called other clinics, explained the urgency for an immediate mammogram. At last, someone listened, understood, and fit her into their schedule for the following day.

That was one of the aggravations of living almost 3,000 miles from Susan while she was going through this trauma. Had I been with her I could have made those phone calls for her and relieved some of her anxiety and frustration.

The evening, after Susan told me she needed a mastectomy, I walked along the shore. It was dusk. The setting sun lent a silver glow to the few clouds in the sky. The craggy rocks looked gray, the water was calm, and I could see the lighthouse emit bright flashes every four seconds. Another wave of emotions encompassed my entire being. My heart was breaking. I cried. As the tide ebbed, so did my anxiety. I knew I would feel that wave again but for a short time, I was at peace.

I arranged flights and traveled cross-country to be with my daughter. At the time, I did not realize she was to have the mastectomy while still receiving chemotherapy. When I learned surgery was needed immediately, I called Bruce. He quickly made airline reservations and flew out to be with us. We needed each other.

We were at the hospital with Susan as she went into surgery for the mastectomy. Once Bruce was able to see how well she was handling all the curves that were thrown her way, he was better able to deal with the reality of what was happening, and found himself in complete agreement with her medical decisions.

Being with Susan helped me a great deal. But then I had to return home. Again, the long distance was difficult but we remained closely connected. Our phone calls and Susan's great sense of humor always gave me a boost. Those waves of emotions continued to catch me off guard. There were times I just could not hold back the tears.

One friend said, "You are not handling this very well at all. Susan is doing a better job than you are."

It was difficult to explain. I thought she would have understood that when a woman's daughter is going through surgery after surgery, it is tough for a mother to hold herself together. I would much rather have been the one undergoing surgery and receiving chemo than to have my daughter in that condition. I believe I could have adjusted to that better than I was able to manage the worry and hurt I felt for Susan.

Other friends were fantastic. Many of them did not know Susan personally but they were still there for me. They repeatedly asked for an update on how Susan was feeling and what treatment she was receiving. Those who did know her, such as one of her former teachers, wanted to know what they could do for Susan. I suggested they simply send a card or write a note to tell Susan they are thinking of her. Little things mean a great deal.

I still could not shake the crashing and ebbing of emotional waves. I felt terribly blue at times, the antithesis of the joy I soaked in when we received good news about Susan's progress.

Kind, caring people provided me support. Support for the support person. The people who understood, or even just tried to understand, what I was going through were the most helpful for me.

I also found strength through research. Reading became a daily occurrence. I read everything I could find relevant to Susan's condition. I wanted to be informed and knowledgeable. I read materials from the local cancer center, the American Cancer Society, and the Susan G. Komen Foundation.

My faith and religious practices were invaluable during this trying time. I felt a connection with a retired monsignor at my church and knew I would be able to talk with him. I went to see him before going to Susan's home on the other side of the country. While telling him about my daughter's diagnosis and what she was encountering physically, I broke down and cried.

With tears still on my face, I said, "Monsignor, I want to be strong when I am with Susan."

With a soft and reassuring tone of voice, he replied, "You will be."

Talking with him gave me strength.

At one point, I said to Susan, "I know you are not big on this 'praying thing' but there are a lot of people who have you in their prayers."

She surprised me when she said, "I've kind of changed on that, Mom. Being in their prayers is sort of nice."

"Get her through this dear God," I pleaded.

Lying in bed one night, I wondered what life would be without Susan. That thought brought another wave, more like a hurricane, of emotion. When I calmed down, I finally slept.

The next morning I thought about others in a state of anxiety. I thought of sources of calmness that could be tapped to ease their journey. Perhaps they could be refreshed by listening to music, reading a book, painting, writing, riding a bike, taking a hike, or just being in their yard surrounded by nature. My personal source was the sight and sound of the ocean.

I walked to the shore. A sense of peace permeated my soul as I felt the rhythm of the surf. I thanked God for Susan's ability to manage her physical adversities, drawing on her own strength and determination. I thanked God for helping me find ways to support my daughter, even though we were thousands of miles apart. I thanked God for the love Susan and I shared; the blessed connection that will never be broken.

Sisters Leap Distance Barriers

We each had magnets on our refrigerators that reminded us to

"Live Well…Laugh Often…Love Much."

During our encounters with cancer, those words became our mantra as we reached out to one another across thousands of miles.

We shared a very special closeness, even though my youngest sister lived in Hawaii, the other in the state of Washington, and I resided in Nevada. Though we were scattered about the far western part of the country, distance could not interfere with our strong bond. We held conference calls at least once a week. We encouraged one another, shared stories about our families, and had the "rah-rah" talks when necessary.

The need for waving our pom-poms seemed to be an ongoing thing. Sandra had heart problems, followed by bladder cancer. Jennifer fought breast cancer for four years, and I was diagnosed with breast cancer. Cancer was prevalent throughout our family, dating back to our grandparents and their relatives. Along the way, Jennifer had additional serious health issues, including ovarian cancer. She was "one tough chic" who was a model of strength and courage.

Through our health challenges, we remained close. The three of us did small things and major things together, even though we were not in the same geographic proximity. For instance, we each collected angels and especially enjoyed giving them to one another. Although we had our weekly calls, we needed to be together. Sandra and I flew across the Pacific to join Jennifer. We shared a glorious week walking on the beach, sitting on the lanai drinking iced tea, talking, and laughing a lot.

We were living our motto: "Live well…laugh often…love much."

The following year we told our husbands we were going to the east coast for a week.

"You just went to Hawaii last year," they said.

We explained in no uncertain terms that they can expect us to continue to reunite at least once a year.

During our second reunion, Jennifer discovered a large hard mass. We cried together. We found humor and laughed together. Jennifer had the mass but Sandra and I shared the pain.

After returning home, we were relieved when Jennifer called to tell us the biopsy revealed the mass was benign. However, all of the radiation she had undergone prevented the tissue from healing. Once again, she took charge. She did research on the internet and found that immense doses of antibiotics could be the cause of her loss of hearing, her knee locking, and her equilibrium being off balance. It took four months, a great deal of suffering, and a lot of sister phone calls, before they changed her treatment. She recovered.

During those months, we walked on a forward-looking path. Jennifer allowed only positives, absolutely no negatives, when we talked to her. We called for test results and simply asked if it was a yes or a no. If it was yes, we were to hang up and give her twenty-four hours to get a grip while we did the same. The next day we discussed what should be done next.

Meanwhile, Sandra continued her fight with bladder cancer. She was treated with chemotherapy and did quite well for ten months. Then it recurred. Once again, off to the chemo chair. Needless to say, we continued lending Sandra strength from a long distance. Our husbands fully understood the high phone bills. They knew those calls were as necessary as food and shelter.

We spent many years providing emotional support for one another. We did not whine about the crosses we had to bear. Even through the tears, we remained positive. We believed that fifty percent of healing is related to attitude.

Positive Attitude

Seven years prior to our cancer encounters, I realized the power of a positive attitude. I lost my first grandson. I cried and I cried and I cried some more. I was on the verge of a nervous breakdown before I became conscious of the fact that I was floundering in a black hole and that crying would not bring back my grandchild.

Jennifer reminded me that it was easier to see in light than in the dark. During the agony of loss and trying times, I remained positive, permitting myself fifteen minutes for pity and tears. My sisters and I allowed each other the same. After one-quarter of an hour of sadness talking about a bad situation, we changed the subject. We shared positive ideas. I found sharing and having an affirmative attitude was a very healthy approach to life's problems.

Almost three years ago, I lost my granddaughter. She was born premature and was not able to survive. I ached for my loss and for my daughter. But I was mentally healthy enough to take hold. I walked down to the pier at the lake. I mourned. My tears flowed from my eyes and my soul. I allowed this to happen for about fifteen minutes and then looked up. I was in awe of the beautiful blue sky, accented with a few puffy clouds. The splendor of the snow-capped mountains, laced with evergreen trees, almost took my breath away. The freshness of the water and fragrance of the evergreen trees added to my feeling of awe. I thanked God for my blessings and for life itself.

Grief is part of loss. We need to release our emotions so we can recover from devastation. However, I would not allow any dark holes or extended periods of time wallowing in sadness. I moved forward and counted my blessings. I believed life is what we choose to make it.

While shopping one day, I spotted a t-shirt that I knew I had to have. In big bold print, it shouted HUG ME. Every time I wore that shirt to the grocery store or just walking down the street, strangers read the words and wrapped their arms around me. That made my day. Most people quickly responded to the message on my shirt, although some were reticent and just smiled.

Those who hugged me said, "Thanks. That felt good."

My sisters and I loved adding rays of sunshine into our worlds. We have been sharegivers, as we called it. Anyone can be a sharegiver/caregiver. Simply open your heart to a person in need.

While growing up, I thought my shoulders were as broad as a man's. My measurements ranged from a 44-inch chest to a 32-inch hip.

I used to tell my friends, "I have broad shoulders. Share your problems with me."

In fact, my nickname throughout high school was Mama because I did so much listening to my friends.

A few years ago, my physician convinced me to have a breast reduction in order to alleviate my back pain.

Afterwards, I looked in the mirror and exclaimed to my husband, "Oh my gosh-I have normal shoulders. They are in proportion with my body."

When I shared that discovery with my girlfriend she replied, "Your shoulders might be normal size but they haven't changed. They are still there when I need to lean on them."

Caregivers often need someone to listen to their thoughts and let them express their emotions. Other times, the mere presence of a friend in silence fills that person's heart and lifts their spirits. Love is what life is all about.

My mantra remains, "Live Well...Laugh Often...Love Much."

One Hundred Fifty Miles from Mom

I left the hospital in a state of denial. I believed there was still plenty of time for the two of us, my mother and me. It was such a shock to find that after five years of being cancer-free, the breast cancer had metastasized and Mom had brain cancer. She immediately began chemotherapy treatments.

Shortly after that horrendous news, Mom was ecstatic when I announced that I was pregnant. She very much wanted a grandchild, so my news left her bursting at the seams with joy. We enjoyed talking about her becoming a grandmother.

She continued treatment and seemed to be doing well. Then, the following April, we learned that Mom's prognosis was terminal.

We lived one-hundred-fifty miles from my parents. I was six months pregnant, and my doctor advised me to stay close to home. He did not want me to travel, especially at seven or eight months. That made it quite difficult for me because I wanted to be with Mom. I talked with my dad and brother often to ask how Mom was doing. I called Mom every day. Talking with her helped me span the miles.

Dad and my brother kept telling me, "Her only wish is that the baby be born healthy."

She knew how sensitive I was so she would not let them tell me what was really going on. Even though Mom was dying, she was concerned about the health and safety of her yet-to-be born grandchild and insisted I see my doctor before driving to Orange County to be with her. To honor Mom's wishes, and for the safety of my baby, I waited until I had my obstetric check-up.

Then it happened quickly.

Dad called. He said, "The doctor told me your mom is not going to be with us much longer."

My husband and I immediately drove down to be with her. A few days later, my entire family insisted I return home for another check-up. They were concerned that my tension about Mom's condition might be affecting the baby. I was reluctant, but we drove home.

Before I was able to get back down to see Mom, she was in a coma. Of course, Dad had not told me in advance, again being protective of our baby. It would have been wonderful if she could have seen her grandchild just once. But that was not to be. However, I know she felt the baby. I was told that when a person is comatose, they can still hear; I talked to Mom. I took her hand and placed it on my stomach. I could actually see her muscles moving and reacting to the feel of her grandchild. I was thankful that she and my unborn child could feel one another.

Mom died April 10; one month to the day, after being told her condition was terminal. She passed on just before Mothers' Day. I cried while I walked the mall shopping for a black maternity dress.

I had not told Mom many of the things I wanted her to know, so I wrote a letter. Not only was my writing a tribute to my mother at her funeral service, it was a great release for me.

It's a Girl!

Seventy days after we lost Mom, our baby was born. It was bittersweet because all Mom wanted was to have a grandbaby. My husband and I did not want to know the sex of our child in advance of its birth, but when I was told the seriousness of Mom's condition, I asked the doctor to tell Mom if she would have a grandson or a granddaughter.

She tried to live long enough to be here for milestones she had written on her calendar. Of course, the baby's birth was one. Another was my baby shower. She was not able to reach those goals but the party-givers followed through with their plans to have the shower.

When I arrived at the hostess' home, everything in the room shouted, "It's a Girl!" Until then, I did not know. I laughed heartily because Mom got the last word! Obviously, she had been excited about the baby and told all of her friends that she would have a granddaughter.

I missed Mom a great deal. I actually felt physical discomfort caused by longing for my mothers presence when my daughter and I did things together. I am grateful that my daughter grew to be like Mom in many ways. Her willpower is a copy of Mom's, she is inquisitive, and she has Mom's initiative.

My mother and I were distanced by 150 miles while she was sick; now we are a world apart. However, our spirits remain entwined.

Words of Wisdom
Long Distance Caregivers

Although it may be heart wrenching to be separated from a person you care about while he or she struggles with a disease, there are things you can do to ease the pain for both of you.

- Let your loved one know you are still there for her or him.

- Call frequently. Hold normal conversations; do not focus on the disease; talk about what is happening with friends and family.

- Play their favorite music over the phone.

- Share sources of calmness that may ease their journey.

- Read aloud poetry or short stories they would enjoy.

- Communicate through e-mail or instant messaging.

- E-mail jokes, funny stories, or pieces of relevant information, such as inspirational messages.

- Arrange for a few of your mutual friends to meet in an electronic chat room.

- Mail surprise packages to your special one. Suggestions include musical CDs, movies, books, crossword puzzles, and easy to handle crafts.

- Send a bouquet of balloons. Have a clown deliver the gift.

- Be alone with thoughts of how special the person is to you. Find solace in fond memories.

2

Expectations

What Should I Expect?

"I was suddenly thrown into the role of a caregiver. I was frightened for Linda and I had no idea what laid ahead or where to turn for help. I wish someone would have given me a few clues about what to expect."

—Randy

I received a call from my former girlfriend just three weeks after we had parted ways. I knew something was wrong. I heard it in her voice. I was not prepared for what she told me.

The news that Linda had breast cancer left me speechless. Cancer took her father's life and she feared the same would happen to her. I found it hard to believe that this was really happening to her. I felt numb. I felt helpless. I wanted desperately to make things right. I'm one who solves problems, straightens out negative situations; but at that time I didn't know what to do or which way to turn. I went to see Linda.

Once I accepted the reality of her condition, I had a strong need to find information about her disease, treatment options and what she might experience—physically and mentally. I talked with cancer patients, caregivers, and health care professionals. By asking questions and listening to many real-life stories, I learned a great deal. I also read books, articles, and searched related websites. I pursued enlightenment about anything relative to her condition. I talked with health care professionals; I asked what physical changes to anticipate during treatment and whether or not she may experience behavioral changes.

My quest for knowledge made me feel empowered; I felt what I was doing would help Linda. I did share my research findings with her. She was sincerely appreciative of my efforts.

The first month following Linda's diagnosis was emotionally difficult for both of us. We were happy with a prognosis report and then dropped to the bottom of the barrel with a conflicting one. Doctors could not be certain of any outcome; all they could do was speculate likelihoods. We were confused and frightened when her oncologist told us things looked grim. Then we were encouraged when the clinical trials health care professional told us that Linda might be a candidate for a new and promising protocol.

We made it through difficult decisions about treatment and, after about four weeks, settled in. We laughed and cried as we felt the peaks and valleys of the roller coaster ride. The connection between us was still alive.

Linda's positive attitude had a lot to do with easing my pain. She was a trooper even when things went wrong often relying on her tremendous sense of humor to make both of us feel better. I learned that caregivers often reflect the attitude of their patient; I certainly did.

To accept reality, I found I needed to process the knowledge I had garnered and the emotions I felt. Cognitively, that worked. I understood the medical procedures involved in her treatment, which was the base of knowledge I needed when I was with her during treatments. I understood intellectually but it took some time to accept it emotionally. She still meant so much to me. Once I overcame my emotional barrier, I was able to move on and be a strong support for Linda.

I was especially grateful for one particular lesson I learned, and later carried into other areas of my life—to live in the moment. Many evenings we laid in Linda's hospital bed together, simply touching, and just being. We were more calm and peaceful than we had ever been because we were not looking at the future. We were truly in the now and were content and happy to be there together.

You Might Anticipate…

Caregivers and victims of any serious disease generally move through psychological phases. They may share these stages, but not necessarily at the same time. These are not clearly defined steps but rather more like riding a horse on a merry-go-round—up, down, round and round, and back again. The process is not mapped out. It is more like a maze. However, know that it does not need to be perplexing. There are others to help you find your way; including other caregivers, counselors, health care professionals, clergy, and friends who have experienced similar circumstances. Be willing to accept help.

Following is Sandra Lahr's description of the psychological stages you might anticipate. Sandra is an oncology nurse and facilitator of a cancer support group.

Shock

Just getting used to the fact that someone you love has a serious disease can be a daunting experience. The grieving process kicks in immediately. It may reveal itself as shock, disbelief, anger, or depression but regardless of the form it takes, grief is normal when a person suffers loss. The diagnosis of a serious disease is a loss of health for the patient and a loss of normalcy in the life of the caregiver.

Disbelief and shock at the time of diagnosis protects the brain for a period of time for all parties involved, until they are able to assimilate the news. This takes longer for some people than others but each person in that initial stage is mentally and emotionally paralyzed until they adjust to the newly acquired information.

From Helplessness to A Quest For Knowledge

In the previous story, once Randy accepted the reality of Linda's condition, he was able to move forward. He began his quest for knowledge, as do many caregivers as they mobilize by conducting extensive research on their loved one's specific disease and types of treatment. Knowledge is power. Randy learned through word of mouth, listening and asking questions. He also read books and articles. He searched the internet for related data. He felt empowered.

Emotional Roller Coaster

Expect the peaks and valleys, much like riding a roller coaster. You may receive good news countered with something not so positive. The ups and downs affect your emotions so don't be surprised if you fluctuate between joy and sadness.

Caregivers often reflect the attitude of their patient. They are so involved with their special person that, without realizing it, they mirror the loved one's mental outlook. If the patient is happy, the caregiver is happy. If he or she is depressed, the caregiver may also feel down. When you become aware of your own behavior and attitude, you are able to take control of your reactions.

Acceptance

Processing knowledge about your loved one's condition will lead to acceptance of the circumstances. At that point, you are better able to evaluate next steps and determine how you will handle the situation.

A Caregiving Police Officer Speaks to Support Groups and Health Care Professionals

I discovered very early in my law enforcement career that one could not predict another's reaction to startling events. The first time I went to a police officer's home to inform his wife that her husband had been killed in the line of duty, I imagined she would collapse into my arms from shock. I was ready for that and knew I could be strong.

Instead, she looked at me and asked, "What will I receive from his insurance?"

I was surprised at her reaction and simply told her I did not have that information but would find the answer for her. The officer's wife remained stoic until her mother walked through the door. At that moment, her apparent numbness subsided and reality set in. She rushed into her mother's open arms and cried hysterically.

A call from my lieutenant sent me to the home of another woman who lost a loved one while he was on duty. When told about his death, she said she wanted to pray and asked if I was Episcopalian.

I replied, "No, but I will pray with you."

She declined, saying she needed to pray with an Episcopalian. Minutes later, my partner arrived. I told him the woman's request.

He whispered, "You are not going to believe this, but there is an Episcopalian Bishop outside in my truck right now."

I was amazed. All I needed to do was listen to the grieving woman and mention her need to someone else. I realized that if we simply open our hearts and ears, the universe will provide.

In the line of duty, I saw tragedy on the streets of the city. I watched cops walk away from the force after they ran head on with a traumatic experience. At the time, they needed to reach out, to talk, to be heard, to cry, and to be comforted; but no one offered.

I learned that such traumas led to an excessive turnover rate of police officers in my city. Three out of five left the force following agonizing occurrences. I related to how those men felt. After serious consideration, I approached my lieutenant with a proposal.

"Let's consider an Employee Assistance Program (EAP) for our traumatized police officers," I suggested. "We can help them; and the budget can be justified because it will reduce employee turnover."

The proposal was accepted. Two of us formed the EAP. Our mission was to provide initial support for officers and their families following a distressful event.

We followed up with appropriate counseling referrals for the officers. Turnover dropped dramatically and, perhaps more importantly, our officers and their families had much needed support.

While continuing to work on the force, I earned a Masters Degree in Contemplative Ministry. I learned not to allow myself to set up behavioral expectations of others. The ministry's approach to interacting with distressed people was to "be there," to be in the present, to listen, observe, and learn how one might help. If we give our full attention to persons in need, they will teach us what to do.

Grief

Dr. Kenneth Doka, a Contemplative Ministry leader, speaks about disenfranchised grief. That is the anguish we, the general public, allow ourselves to grieve if a spouse or mother dies, but we do not allow ourselves to be sad if our pet dies or best friend moves to another town. I cannot emphasize strongly enough, how important it is to be in the present for others, regardless of how you may perceive the depth of their loss.

Two Steps of Grieving

People grieve for different lengths of time and on varying levels. Psychologists have espoused a number of theories about grief. I share with you the two steps I experienced when my dad died.

First, I was angry. Throughout the years, I knew my dad loved me, but it had been a long distance relationship after I moved from home to attend school in another town. I wish I had known my dad better. He died at the age of sixty-nine. I did not have the opportunity to ask him many questions. After his death, I wondered what he would have thought of our presidents, if he had any prejudices, or how he would feel about his grandchildren. I was angry because he was gone.

The second step, acceptance, was critical for me. I knew I could not change the loss of my father but acceptance of his death allowed me to have control over my life and feelings. I reconciled the fact that he was not here to see me receive my bachelors or masters degree, to see my children, or to enjoy retirement with me. I accepted reality.

Support Groups

Support groups were not available when I initiated an Employee Assistance Program for police officers. The EAP was a wonderful source of comfort and direction for the officers and their families but now I know they could have drawn extra strength from being part of a support group. Sharing feelings and thoughts about stressful situations acts as a pressure valve, releasing pent up emotions and concerns. Sharing with people who have been or presently are in similar circumstances also provides learning opportunities regarding specific problems.

Our Paths Vary

I retired from the police force. I practice Contemplative Ministry, teaching others to be in the present. One of my great joys is speaking to support groups, doctors, nurses, and other health care professionals, about listening to and learning from someone in need. Healing is more than a physical process. Human beings also need attention given to their emotional, psychological, and spiritual needs as well. A holistic approach to healing has proven to be a beneficial means of treatment.

Whether or not you belong to a support group, you can be a wonderful caregiver. Please know that you do not need a Ph.D. You do not need a Masters or a Bachelors Degree. You simply need to be someone who listens, has an open heart, and is willing to be in the present to learn what others need, not what you expect of him or her.

Listen and you will learn. Learn and you will be rewarded with the glorious feeling of knowing you have made a difference in someone's life.

Words of Wisdom
Expectations and Grief

- Be ready for change.
- Ask the medical team what to expect in the way of physical and behavioral changes in your patient.
- Knowledge is power. Research your loved one's disease, including physical and behavioral changes that may occur.
- Caregivers personally experience change within themselves and in their daily lives. Personal adjustments one may face include disruption in your daily routine, riding an emotional roller coaster, discovery of the depth of love you feel for your patient, or you may face the fight or flight syndrome.

- Reach out for help. Counselors, support groups, social workers, and health care professionals can help you make decisions that are right for you. Know that seeking help is not a sign of weakness—it is a sign of strength. Recognize your internal and external sources of strength; tap on them for support.

- Family members still need you but you discover you do not have much energy left for them. Do not feel guilty. Do talk with them, especially children, and together develop a plan that will meet their needs, as well as yours. Help them differentiate between needs and desires. Ask them to understand that things will be different for a while.

- Expect seemingly unyielding demands on your time. Be prepared and willing to ask for help.

- Financial challenges may crop up as you pay medical bills. Research sources of financial aid.

- Make decisions about how you will best spend your energy. You can wear a superman costume on Halloween; avoid the urge to do so in your daily life.

3

Relationships

COPING WITHIN RELATIONSHIPS
by Sandra Lahr

As an oncology nurse and facilitator in a cancer center, I've had the opportunity to work closely with caregivers. Each situation is different with every individual who comes in for medical evaluation and treatment. The same holds true for caregivers. However, there are also similarities.

Using their own coping mechanisms, people connected through kinship or friendship have already dealt with the waxing and waning of problems or crises amongst themselves. When a diagnosis of cancer or any other serious disease enters into the bond they share, all of the things that had previously been in play will continue after the illness is identified. Some will be good and some not as healthy as one would hope.

Fortunately, we've seen a great deal of positive coping by those in a healthy relationship. The caregiver is devastated, in many ways the same as their loved one, by the news that their special person has a serious disease. The depth of the heartache can be even greater for the caregiver than that of the patient. You may wonder how that could be possible. It's because the caregiver feels absolutely helpless to change the situation. Love accentuates the pain but it also motivates people to act.

Primary caregivers are often passionate in their search for new knowledge about their loved one's disease and potential treatments. They learn all they can on their own. They become obsessed in their quest for information. They view their research efforts as one way to help that person back to good health or perhaps sooth their journey as they move towards a peaceful death. In the process, they increase their own stamina because, as we know, there is strength in knowledge. Knowledge is power.

They both learn new ways of coping, which helps to dispel the anxieties and fears that come with the diagnosis of a serious disease right from the beginning. For instance, by seeking knowledge they gain a reprieve from anxiety and fears that otherwise may be overwhelming. They face it all head-on as they work through the crisis. In the process, their connection deepens and they know they can face the crisis together.

We often see each of them journaling as they move through this difficult experience. It becomes their obsession, their mission, to express their love. It is a beautiful thing to see caregivers and patients create books for one another.

However

Unfortunately, there are situations where people simply cannot cope with the diagnosis of serious disease or disability in their family. My colleagues and I have seen those relationships break up. We've seen estrangement from children to parent; we've seen husbands leaving wives and wives leaving husbands. Sometimes that's all the relationship needed for it to dissolve. That is the ultimate sadness in crisis but we also know that sometimes it's just the evolution of life and out of that comes new and beautiful things, maybe for all involved.

Coping

Certainly when it comes to family, we see different coping mechanisms within that connected group of people. For instance, in terms of adult children and a parent, some children are able to cope very well; others may not be able to deal with their parent's diagnosis so they withdraw and turn the responsibility over to their siblings who are able to meet the crisis. If one person feels like they're carrying the brunt of it all because a sister or brother is unable to cope, that may create new divisions within the family.

From the nursing perspective, we embrace the entire family. We try to help the family by working with each person concerning their own issues, assisting them in dealing with the crisis that has come into their lives.

Caregivers' Reactions and Responsibilities

The primary caregiver's initial reaction to the loved one's diagnosis of a serious disease is to think, "She or he has it far worse than I do. I need to be stoic and strong."

The reality is that the caregiver is also in crisis. It's not just the patient who is suffering. Caregivers need to be reminded of this and be given support. They may feel they suddenly have to carry the ball alone as they help their loved one with health care needs and shore up the family. It's very likely that they also assume additional responsibilities because the patient is overwhelmed with doctors' appointments, receiving treatment, feeling weak and tired and unable to handle even the simplest tasks around the house. The person with the diagnosis may have been a wage earner for the household and now the total financial burdens fall upon the caregiver.

Other responsibilities may include housekeeping, grocery shopping, laundry, and paying the bills. The list of action items seems to grow daily; solving insurance problems, driving the patient to and from the doctor's office, or being there in a nursing capacity to help with his or her basic physical needs or medical attention. If children are involved, childcare needs to be arranged; if aging parents require guardianship that also may become the primary caregiver's responsibility. All of this, at the cost of the caregiver's own well-being.

Yet the mechanism of adrenalin kicks in and people do what they have to do; certainly, when there is a love component, they have strength they didn't realize they could possibly possess within themselves.

Interaction between Caregiver and Patient

In relationships, many crises occur every day. But when one feels he or she can't burden the other person with these problems, new stressors are likely to develop between the two people. Frustrations grow simply because the caregiver is working through exhaustion and has ignored his or her own needs. This is common in these situations because it is done out of love. But the caregivers need to be reminded that their own needs must be maintained while tending to their loved one. Everyone has a breaking point and a caregiver cannot provide the good-intentioned support for their loved one if she or he insists on carrying the entire load alone. They must ask for help.

We also know that how the patient copes with his or her situation is often reflected by the caregiver. If he or she uses a negative coping style, the caregiver may become a mirror to that type of survival technique. On the other hand, if the patient is coping very well, his caregiver is able to be more open to his or her own feelings and frustrations. By addressing these issues, the door opens for enhanced communication and understanding between the two of them. It reinforces their belief that they can get through this together.

Coping Mechanisms

A crucial medical diagnosis hits the family hard. As with any trauma, people are in a state of shock and reach back to coping mechanisms they have garnered along the way. Some of the methods are healthy ways of dealing with stress. Others are not. There are those who turn to excessive alcohol consumption, using drugs, kicking the dog, slamming doors…none of which is a healthy means of handling stress. However, there are innumerable healthy coping mechanisms.

As nurses, we have the responsibility to help patients and caregivers recognize how they are coping and possibly introduce new means of handling stress. But opening the stress control tool box and pulling out generic techniques is not the answer. The coping style must fit the person.

We help them identify their key stressors. A significant one may be fear of losing their loved one but at the moment, the major stressor may be simply adjusting to disruption of their day-to-day life style. Learning how to care for their sick one may be difficult; or prioritizing all that needs to be accomplished may seem overwhelming.

As nurses, we get to know these caregivers so we are better able to guide them. We help select the appropriate coping mechanisms from those they've used in the past or other methods we may suggest. They determine what will work for them. It could be as simple as taking a walk every afternoon or as complex as needing to learn how to take care of their loved one's physical needs. If the myriad of methods we discuss don't work, the door is always open for further guidance.

As a caregiver, you probably already know your loved one's personality, needs and how to help them consider variable coping mechanisms. If not, I encourage you both to talk with a counselor, religious or spiritual guide, or anyone who can help you identify your stressors and determine how to alleviate some of the tension.

Breaking Point

There are times caregivers can give with every ounce of energy they have. However, they need to recognize their own limitations when they feel drained and need to find a way to regroup, relax, and rejuvenate.

People in these intense situations may be handling everything in an ostensibly calm manner but are churning inside. They may be surprised at their own behavior when, suddenly, anger lashes out. Then they feel badly about losing their temper. It is important to understand that emotions build and fluctuate. We ask caregivers to be alert for warning signs, those signals that indicate their emotional state. Perhaps they're feeling irritable, exhausted, or withdrawn. If they can identify their own symptoms, they're more likely to be able to take action to alleviate the tension before they reach a breaking point.

When the Oxygen Mask Drops

Flight attendants tell passengers, "If you're traveling with someone who needs assistance, adjust your oxygen mask before helping the other person."

Those are wise words of advice. You may be inclined to want to help your loved one before yourself but if you do, you risk losing your own strength when it is needed most.

Take care of yourself!

CAREGIVING HUSBANDS

Big Boys Don't Cry

"Cancer is not about one person suffering. Cancer is about each of us. It is a disease that affects us all."

—Bob Ginsberg

First-time patients in a doctor's office always complete voluminous pages of a medical history questionnaire. I think we have completed reams of paper work since Judi was diagnosed with breast cancer.

At various times in my life, I have entered my medical history on doctors' forms.

The questions always included, "Has anyone in your family been diagnosed with cancer?'"

I answered yes, a resounding yes. Direct line. My dad, my brother—cancer took their lives. I thought it was likely I would be next.

Judi and I discussed that possibility many times during our thirty-five years together. We knew how to communicate! We talked and we listened to one another. We spoke openly about the possibility of my life being cut short by cancer, prevalent in my family history. But the shocker was that Judi, my wonderful wife, was the one diagnosed with cancer, the disease I feared. She had breast cancer—stage four. I could not believe it.

I kept asking myself, "Why Judi, why? Cancer was not in her family, it was in mine."

My brother, Joe, was diagnosed with the same disease that had taken my dad. When Joe learned he had cancer, he decided that it would take his life. But I did not find his attitude the least bit acceptable. Many days, I traveled an hour and a half each way to be with Joe while he was undergoing treatment. I talked with him until I was hoarse. I tried to convince him that because Dad died from cancer did NOT mean he needed to do the same.

Joe consistently retorted, "Dad died from cancer. So will I. That's how it will be."

I continued to try to persuade Joe to make an effort towards getting well. He was finally convinced. He wanted to win the battle. When he told me he wanted to live, I cried tears of joy. But the tears and love could not wash away the fact that Joe had waited too long. His body no longer had the strength to be victorious in his struggle for life.

Having gone through those difficult times with my dad and brother, it was especially tough for me to face the fact that Judi needed to encounter ongoing tests, surgery, and chemotherapy. Judi was the love of my life; I hurt for her.

Then I thought, "This is <u>our</u> cancer. I can't protect her from the disease but I can provide strong, unwavering support."

I knew in my heart that we could overcome this adversity together. We would take on the challenge as a couple. One of my key jobs would be to make her laugh.

Humor was an integral part of our relationship. I believed laughter would help heal Judi's body.

Our motto was, "Keep a smile on your face and approach the enemy with a positive attitude. Laugh! Just do it!"

I supported Judi in every way possible. We went to medical appointments and attended support group meetings together. We traveled to Houston for Judi's treatments at M.D. Anderson Cancer Center. At home, I prepared food, cleaned house, and made her laugh!

Judi was concerned about having a mastectomy and talked with me about the outcome of that procedure.

I said, "Judi, all you are giving up is cancer."

Then she wanted my opinion on her having breast reconstruction.

I said, "Judi, I love you far beyond appearance. You need to make that decision for yourself. You must do what will make you feel best about yourself. I love you for what you are inside, not your physical appearance."

She chose not to have reconstruction.

As we traveled the hilly road together, I remained strong. I stayed by my wife's side, making her laugh, and raising her spirits when they began to droop. Judi called me her "rock."

I thought I was holding up well. Then I realized I was behaving differently. I projected myself out of my body, I saw myself across the room. I became aware that I didn't care about anything—not my job, not my kids, not my family—nothing, except Judi. I knew I needed to seek help.

I talked to Judi. I explained that her "rock" was crumbling. I did not want to burden her with another problem but I needed to talk. Communication was part of our strength as a couple. I needed her support. She listened intently and understood how I was feeling.

Then she asked, "What are you going to do, Bob?"

I answered, "I'm not sure."

Two days later, my boss told our employee group we now had an EAP, an Employee Assistance Plan. Counselors were available to discuss any of our needs. That was my answer. I decided to talk with one of the EAP therapists.

Listless

I explained to the counselor that I was listless and did not care about anything but Judi getting well. I had no energy and did not want to go to work. My laughter had subsided and I viewed that as a symptom of a serious problem.

"I have always been like a brick wall—until Judi's diagnosis," I told the counselor. I said, "Judi's rock is crumbling into pebbles. I've always backed Judi, but now I don't have the strength I need at the time she needs me most."

The EAP therapist talked with me about my symptoms.

He said, "People experience depression and listlessness while facing challenges and trauma. Be reassured that things WILL improve. You are having very normal reactions to the stress and anxiety you are experiencing."

Two weeks later, I returned to the counselor's office. I was feeling much better and wanted to thank him for his help.

I returned to work, even though a few weeks earlier I did not think I could muster up enough energy to handle my job. However, I had changed. I talked about cancer with everyone I met. I told the young people at work about the disease and how it affects the victim's family and friends. I no longer kept my problems to myself. I released them. I received wonderful support; and by sharing my problems, I believe many people learned something about coping with adversity.

Life changes when a serious disease enters the door of life. I'm not sure my life will ever be the same as it was before Judi's diagnosis, but some changes are for the best. I came out of our cancer battle with an entirely different perspective of life and people. Patients often say they feel stronger after winning the battle against this disease. Caregivers feel the same.

As a young lad I was taught that "Big boys don't cry." As a grown man, I've learned that not only do big boys cry...real men weep.

It's No Big Deal

As a child, I was taught to be helpful, to lend a hand wherever needed, whether it was for my parents, friends, relatives or others who might need assistance. As I grew into manhood, I continued to help others. To me, it was just the right thing to do. I never gave it a second thought. Others cared for me when I was sick or feeling down and I did the same for them. I helped through childbirth, raising a family, aided ill and dying parents, and still thought this was all just part of life. "No big deal."

When my wife and I first met, I knew she was a loving and caring person. She was always available to help people through their day-to-day troubles and problems. She was a good listener and a mentor. I knew we shared an important value—that of caring for others.

While we were dating, she encountered some physical problems. I was there to help when she broke her wrist, injured her ankle, had knee surgery and a hysterectomy.

I did what I could to ease her back to health, all the time thinking, "No big deal. I can do this."

Six years after we were married, Peg told me she discovered a lump on her breast and planned to see a doctor. Just three years earlier, her sister had been treated for breast cancer. My wife was taking no chances. The surgeon arranged for a mammogram. Next, he surgically removed breast tissue. The procedures did not reveal any abnormalities. That was good news. Another "no big deal."

But the lump increased in size. The surgeon recommended a lumpectomy. We were off to the hospital, once again. My first thoughts were to be very supportive but not let her know that I was troubled about this new development. I did not want her to be concerned about me. I felt she needed to muster all the strength she could for the surgery. I tried to remain calm.

But I no longer could say, "It's no big deal."

When I first began to think this could lead into a serious problem I told myself to think of our grandson, who would have said, "No way, Grandpa!"

We arrived at the hospital very early on the appointed day. The prep took less than thirty minutes. Then the waiting began. An hour and a half later, Peg was wheeled on a gurney to the surgical area. I was told the procedure should not take more than forty-five minutes and that I would know how she was doing within the hour.

It was pretty much an exercise in futility, but I did try to work word puzzles to keep my mind occupied. I was worried. Forty-five minutes passed, then an hour. After an hour and a half of fidgeting and pacing, I still had heard nothing. Finally, I saw her surgeon walking towards me.

My heart skipped a couple of beats, not knowing what to expect.

He said, "Peg went through the procedure without any problems. She is in the recovery unit and you can go see her. Oh, by the way, sorry about the delay in telling you. I was running late so there was a forty-five minute delay in beginning the procedure."

I was extremely relieved that she was alright, but I wondered why no one had kept me informed. Hospital staff need to be aware of the person waiting for information; they must know how stressful it is for caregivers to wait beyond the anticipated period planned for procedures.

I rushed to recovery. I felt much better when I could see and hold her. Four days later, I was at work when my office phone rang. I could tell the moment I answered that something was terribly wrong.

Peg said, "Dr. Samuel called with the biopsy results. I have cancer."

Nothing in the world could have prepared me for this.

Again, I told myself, "Be strong. Don't let on that you are worried."

As though she would not know. Ha! She knew me well. But, she was strong and let me pretend to be worry-free, even though I knew she could see right through that facade.

For the next several weeks things were really rough. We were already in the process of preparing to relocate to another state when she received the diagnosis. I encouraged her to have the surgery and treatment done before we moved but Peg wanted to move forward with life. Relocation was in that plan. We proceeded with all that goes with a long distance move, the entire time having another surgical procedure and follow-up treatment on our minds. The move was our third in six years. We had become pros and I believed everything would go smoothly.

"No way, Grandpa."

We encountered major problems with the builder and the moving company. A week after we moved into the new house one of our cats disappeared. Just what we needed. More stress.

But we kept moving forward. Peg had her first medical appointment in our new location the day the movers were carrying furniture into the house. During the following ten days she spent most of her time making medical appointments, talking with our health insurance provider, seeing specialists, and unpacking boxes.

Surgery was scheduled. We were back to the hospital. Once again Peg was taken into the operating room and remained there almost three times as long as they had told me to expect. My worrying increased and I started asking myself some serious questions that had never crossed my mind.

I wondered, "How will I tell her daughter what has happened? Should I call Jack, her son, first so he can tell Katie? And how about Judy and Lin, her sisters? Should I call my daughters first so I have their support? Where will I turn? I'm a stranger in a new town. I'm alone. What will I do if something serious happens? Family will take a while to get here. What if she dies? Does she really want me to follow the wishes of her will? We have not talked about that for years. Maybe she's changed her mind."

My thoughts were swimming. My heart was aching.

The new surgeon appeared.

He said, "The cancer was much deeper than I anticipated. I had to perform a partial mastectomy; her left breast will be one inch smaller than her right, but I expect her to fully recover."

I was greatly relieved. Nothing else mattered as long as Peg would be here to love and share life with me.

I did not realize how uptight I was feeling but when I walked through the hospital doors to the parking lot, I stopped. It dawned on me that I had no idea where I parked our car. I searched the parking lot. Meanwhile, a nurse's aide stood with my wife as she sat in a wheel chair and waited to be picked up. Peg knew I would eventually show up but was worried that something was wrong. When I explained what happened, we both laughed. She fully understood. We left the hospital and drove home.

A few days later we heard the good news. The surgeons were able to remove the cancer cells. She needed radiation but not chemotherapy. She recovered wonderfully.

I have been blessed to have few traumatic experiences in my life. However, I must be straightforward. Peg's cancer threat scarred the hell out of me. My compassion goes out to anyone experiencing such an ordeal. **It is a big deal!**

My Husband—My Mainstay

Derek was my mainstay. I could not have gone through double mastectomies and months of chemotherapy without my dear husband's love and support.

He found it difficult to see me in pain, but I think facing his fear of what the future might hold was extremely frightening. He did everything possible to help me. He knew I wasn't satisfied with the clinic where the diagnosis had been made. I made an appointment at the City of Hope, even though it was fifty-five miles from home. I felt safe and secure there so he agreed to change to that medical facility.

After our first appointment at the City of Hope, he said, "Don't worry about the hour-long drive. You need to be here."

He changed his work schedule to accommodate all of my medical appointments; every single one. He was with me for chemotherapy treatments, appointments with the oncologist, plastic surgeon and the gynecologist. I regained my strength and returned to work. When Derek had questions, he accompanied me to meetings with various health care professionals. He was incredibly supportive and approached everything with a positive attitude. I worked in the medical field so I was very aware that cancer could recur.

But Derek, from the moment I came out of surgery, said "You are now cancer free. You will remain cancer free."

He continued to believe that, which helped me look at it through his optimistic eyes.

He and I have always communicated well. During my battle with cancer, I discovered I needed to talk about my fears. I told him I was afraid. I asked what he thought the doctors would find or what he thought would happen. He remained positive. He went to the first few follow-up appointments just because he knew I was still frightened.

I asked myself, "What will I do if I am at the City of Hope without Derek and the doctor tells me I have a recurrence?" I answered my own question. "It's not going to happen so why worry."

We talked. We laughed. We prayed.

Derek and I found that our faith was our source of strength. The night I was told that cancer was in both breasts, we were stunned and frightened. Our pastor and a very good friend came to our house. Reverend Bob talked to me while our friend, Sam, talked to Derek. Then we all prayed together. Our minister gave me two very short prayers to recite over and over when I needed comfort.

The first was one line, "Lord Jesus Christ, have mercy on me."

The second was from the book of Psalms; "Be still and know that I am God."

Those two short phrases provided me with much comfort, peace and strength.

Derek joined a men's group at church. That provided him an open door to share his thoughts, feelings, and fears with other men who were understanding and gave him strength. I continued my involvement with the women's covenant group at church and drew inspiration from those wonderful ladies.

My husband and I shared our faith, which helped shore us both up. I thank God for my dear husband, my mainstay, as we sailed the rocky waters of cancer treatment.

Rose Petals

A simple tonsillectomy, that's all. I told myself not to worry. But as I sat in the surgical waiting room I couldn't help but be concerned because my dear Rose was undergoing surgery. Then I saw her surgeon walking toward me. As I stood to meet him, I noticed that he seemed to be in a hurry.

His voice conveyed urgency when he said, "I must talk with you. Your wife's tonsils were removed successfully but I discovered a large mass behind those lymphoid tissues. It is critical that we take action immediately."

That same day, we went to the imaging clinic where Rose had a C.A.T. scan. One week later she was in surgery for removal of the suspicious lump.

The biopsy revealed a malignant growth. I was devastated to know that Rose had cancer. However, I was determined to be strong, mentally and emotionally, for Rose. I kept a positive attitude as she and I discussed what steps to take next.

Rose's dad called and asked to speak to me. Her family lived on the east coast and they wanted her to come home for treatment at Sloan Kettering, the medical facility that is world famous for successful cancer treatment. We were in full agreement. Within a week, her family made all of the arrangements. We flew to New York.

My boss and coworkers were fantastic. They supported me all the way, encouraging me to stay in New York as long as was necessary. We were there five weeks. At that time, her oncologist told us she could receive the same treatment in the city where we lived. We returned home.

Rose and I had always communicated freely and she expected, rightly so, for that to continue while we fought this disease. After we were told her cancer was incurable, I slipped in and out of denial. She tried to talk with me about the reality of the situation.

She said, "There are certain things we need to discuss."

I listened and understood what she was saying, but that was not easy. Regardless of the gravity of the situation, I vowed to move forward and do all I could to make her happy.

One evening I overheard Rose telling friends, "My husband manages to keep his positive attitude as we encounter daily ups and downs. He's very good at making me laugh, even after one of those 'We need to talk' conversations. He has a way of making me feel better when things look bleak."

The roller coaster ride intensified. Good news—the cancer seemed to be in remission. Bad news—it had metastasized to her lungs. Good news—she could participate in clinical trials. Bad news—that didn't work. We needed to try something else. As we followed all leads, Rose maintained a positive but realistic approach to the status of her health.

We joined a cancer support group and attended weekly meetings. We both learned a lot from patients AND their caregivers. Perhaps the greatest gift was the strength we gained from those wonderful, compassionate, and loving people. They told Rose innumerable times that she brought sunshine and hope to others. Her positive attitude was contagious. She was indeed loved. The evening she announced the cancer had metastasized to her lungs, people cried.

The fragrance and velvet-soft petals of my dear Rose began to lose their color. She was tired. She knew her condition was terminal and accepted that reality. She even met with a priest and planned her own funeral.

A friend I had met at the support group forewarned me that I would feel pain and need support. He had been through the same thing with his first wife. He encouraged me to reach out for support.

I was determined to be strong but the time did come when I knew my friend was right. I had support from the group and, of course, from Rose. My family called frequently. Rose's mom and brother flew to see Rose as soon as they heard the disease had also attacked her lymph nodes. Her dear niece traveled cross-country to be with her. Rose's sister, friends, and family came from near and far. They all wanted to be with Rose.

It is not easy for men to cry in front of anyone and I certainly did not want to break down in front of Rose. But with her brother, it happened. As we talked, I suddenly burst into tears. I sobbed, tried to catch my breath and control the tears. But once the flood gates opened, I couldn't stop. Her brother cried with me. It was a catharsis for both of us. When we regained our composure we talked more about losing Rose.

I also talked one on one with a couple of men from the support group. I found that very helpful.

Over and over I told Rose how much I loved her. As the days slipped by my heart was breaking. I knew she would soon be gone from me and from this earth.

The priest she had come to know as she planned her own funeral became her friend. He officiated at her memorial service. Friends and family filled the church. As a final tribute to my beautiful Rose, the congregation gathered in front of the church after the service. We released white doves into the heavens. Rose was now pain free and at peace. My beautiful flower left gardens of love in the hearts of family and many, many friends. She will always bloom within my soul.

Words of Wisdom
Caregiving Husbands

"You can't protect your wife from disease but you can help her through a difficult struggle."

—Bob Ginsberg

A man caring for his ailing wife may find himself doing many things to relieve her anxiety, including accompanying her to medical appointments, comforting her as the two of you sit quietly together—just being in the moment, busily cleaning the house, or tending to her physical needs. The following words of wisdom are the lessons men learned while being the primary persons who cared for their wives.

- Take on the challenge together, as a couple.

- Keep humor alive in your relationship. Laughter is superb medicine.

- Communicate with her. Share your feelings and thoughts about what is happening, helping to keep both of you balanced.

- Eliminate the word stoic from your vocabulary. Yes, you are strong. Yes, you can do this. However, it is essential that you recognize and accept the fact that, as a caregiver, you need support from others.

- Reach out to friends, family, counselors, and support groups.

- Take care of yourself! That means emotionally, spiritually, and physically. You need your strength. Make time for yourself: exercise, play golf, bowl, read a book—whatever gives you pleasure and leaves you feeling rejuvenated.

WOMEN CARING FOR THEIR MEN

My Number One Priority

Did I consider myself a caregiver as I walked out of the hospital with Joe? No. I hadn't even given that a thought. I had no idea what laid ahead; how my life would change.

Joe and I had lived the past thirty-six years doing almost everything together. We married, raised children, and shared responsibilities for our family business. Our lives were closely intertwined, although we did have our individual activities. We loved one another and the life we had built together.

In our fifties, we both developed arthritis but Joe's was more severe than mine. He had surgery to fuse bones in his ankle. He spent six weeks in a cast, three weeks using crutches to ambulate and then he was back into the molded plaster around his ankle. During the last six weeks in a cast, he rubbed open the skin on his heel.

One Sunday morning, he put his weight on his left heel as he was getting out of the car after church. He complained of pain. When I looked at his foot I noticed his toe was inflamed. Joe insisted that we wait to see the doctor at his scheduled appointment on Tuesday. I balked at that idea but acquiesced to his wishes.

I took him to see the orthopedic specialist, as planned. Joe described the pain in his heel but the doctor was not the least bit concerned.

He said, "Perhaps it's just a heel spur."

I told him that Joe had been running a fever for the past few days but Dr. Larry still didn't perceive any problem.

It was time to be more than assertive. I had to become aggressive. I absolutely insisted that he contact our primary care physician immediately. He did so; although he seemed reluctant and still thought there was nothing to worry about.

As we drove to Dr. Ray's diagnostic center, Joe commented on my aggressiveness. He was surprised I was so demanding, even though he understood that I was seriously troubled about his condition and would not let anything slide by us. He told me he didn't feel bold and ready to pursue the subject because he did not want to go to the hospital.

As it turned out, he had no choice. Dr. Ray examined Joe and sent him straight to the hospital, where the nurse drew fluid from Joe's heel. Then an infectious disease specialist was called in to diagnose Joe's condition. He prescribed antibiotics to combat staph infection. The doctor explained that people with rheumatoid arthritis are more susceptible to staph infection because their immune system is weak. Later, I told the orthopedic specialist about the connection between the two. That bit of information finally commanded his attention.

A Picc line was placed in Joe's chest so that, while he was home, he could receive antibiotics intravenously. The nurse showed me how to administer the medications and trained me to change the bag without exposing the line. I was told to call if I had any problem.

During those six weeks, Joe stopped taking all of his arthritic medications to prevent any interference with the antibiotics. As a result, his entire body was racked with pain. I was there to give him the urinal when needed. He was unable to shower so I bathed him and handed him his toothbrush, tooth paste, razor and shaving cream. He sat by the bathroom sink to shave and care for his dental hygiene.

He had difficulty sleeping and I wanted to be quick to respond if he needed something. I considered sleeping in bed with a baby monitor nearby so I could hear his movements. I decided against that. I wanted to be close to him so I slept on a pallet of blankets placed on the floor next to his bed.

After many years of Joe taking prescribed drugs, suddenly I was responsible for giving him his meds. I assumed the role of a nurse without having the medical knowledge. But that technical information was just a phone call away if I had inquiries.

My life changed as I became consumed with caring for Joe. As I did everything for him, other responsibilities had to be put aside. He was my absolute number one priority and I had to learn to leave many things undone. In our office, bills sat on my desk unpaid. At home, the utility room filled with laundry. I remember the day I left breakfast dishes setting on the table because I wanted to get outside early to plant a garden for Joe. He loved to grow tomatoes, beans, corn, and potatoes. I wanted that garden for him, hoping it would give him pleasure while he was sick.

There were times when the backlog of tasks bothered me but I learned to simply take things as they came my way. I needed to let go of the desire to be on top of things; running an office and a home efficiently just was not going to happen while I cared for Joe.

He was a wonderful patient who was grateful for all acts of kindness. Joe often told me how much he appreciated my caring for his medical, physical, and even emotional needs. His appreciation warmed my heart and was an incentive to keep going even when I felt exhausted.

Although those several months were difficult, Joe and I had good times together. Our communication rose to a new level. We told one another things we had never said before. He talked about how much I have always meant to him and I shared my deep feelings for him. We even renewed our wedding vows—without a ceremony.

We realized that because we were together constantly, at home and work, taking one another for granted had become our modus operandi. That changed. We made a point of taking time to share our thoughts and feelings.

Music played an important role in Joe's life, so while he was sick it was only natural that he listened to melodies and symphonies. When either one of us needed calmness I played the CD from the movie, *Pretty Horses*. Joe cried. I cried. We both felt better.

I recalled that while Joe's cousin was seriously ill, she was soothed by playing musical tapes that included varying gentle sounds, such as waves lapping on the shore, wind rustling through the trees, or birds singing. Joe and I found the same to be true for both of us.

Throughout the several months of our ordeal, our friends were magnificent. They brought meals, stopped to visit, sent cards to both of us, e-mailed messages of support, and recommended books that might be helpful. I considered those supportive people very important! Knowing there were others who cared about us gave me inner strength.

That stamina remained with me. Perhaps it was because of my Christian faith. When I had dark moments I'd ask God for inner strength; it was provided. And when I prayed for physical strength in my arthritic hands so I could give Joe the massages he needed, my prayers were answered.

I think that life prepares us for adversity. Losing my mother at a young age, Joe's dad passing on, and the loss of three of his closest friends in a very short period of time, were extremely difficult. In retrospect, I know I grew with each of those happenings.

Joe's health improved significantly. We were able to go to football and basketball games again. I learned how to use disability access, ramps and wheelchairs. We resumed our lives with altered approaches to our daily tasks. We grew together and adjusted to the challenges of rheumatoid arthritis. I resumed some of my activities, singing in the church choir and teaching Sunday school.

Most importantly, we were grateful for each other, our family, and our friends. Our love abounds for all.

Persistent and Grateful

Ken said, "I don't need to worry. You do enough for both of us."

That may have been true but when he was diagnosed with cancer, I was deeply concerned. The first doctor who looked at the acorn-sized knot on his tongue told him not to worry. I insisted he see my dentist, who immediately sent him to an oncologist. Not only was the lump malignant, it was classified as stage-four cancer because it had metastasized into his lymph nodes.

When I heard the diagnosis, I couldn't hold back the tears. I was scared. I didn't want to lose Ken. We had been together for several years and I loved him dearly.

He wanted to believe there was nothing upsetting about this latest news. I was sure he was covering his real feelings. Eighteen years earlier, his wife died from cancer. I knew he was reliving some of that grief and fear.

To make matters worse, he had diabetes at the time he was diagnosed with cancer. Then he had a mild stroke.

"How much more can his body handle?" I asked myself.

We found the answer to that question after he had surgery that lasted thirteen hours. I walked into the recovery room and gasped. With so many drains in his body he looked like an octopus. However, he improved daily and I was amazed at his marvelous progress.

During all of this, I asked many questions of his health care team. I did not have much success finding answers about his condition, probably because we were not married and they did not want to divulge personal information. I asked Ken to question the doctors but he was not comfortable doing so. I continued my quest for information. I conducted research on the internet, at the library, and called the American Cancer Society. I asked questions of my dentist, my primary care physician, and people I met that had been treated for tongue cancer.

That was an amazing thing. As I began to bring tongue cancer into my conversations with friends, they told me of survivors they knew who had been successfully treated for the same disease. I called anyone willing to talk with me. One man I spoke with had been told that continuing radiation treatment was not an option; surgery was the only answer. He revolted.

In no uncertain terms, he said, "I will not have my tongue cut from my mouth!"

He and his wife were aggressive in their search to find other opinions. They were fortunate to be able to go to M.D. Anderson, an esteem cancer center in Houston. That trip led to an alternate treatment which saved his tongue—and his life.

I continued to hear about how important it was for the patient and caregiver to be assertive; to take charge of whatever was necessary to obtain the best treatment. I found that it was often the caregivers who did the research, made the phone calls, and then shared the information with their patient. That is a plus, not just for the person who has a disease, but for the caregiver who feels he or she is able to do something of value to help.

We lived in a small town fifty miles from the hospital where Ken had surgery and received treatment. His sister and brother-in-law lived in the city, not far from that medical facility. They opened their home and their hearts to us. We stayed with them for several weeks. What a God-send they were with their love, understanding and hospitality. During our stay, they welcomed our friends who came to visit Ken. The dear people who stopped by were a blessing, as were those who called, sent cards and shared information. The friends, acquaintances and family who supported us, regardless of the extent of their level of involvement with Ken and I, played a critical role in helping us through a challenging epic in our lives. We were fortunate to have such support.

Words of Wisdom
Women Caring For Their Men

When your loved one is diagnosed with disease, or incapacitated in some way, caring for him becomes your number one priority. The following advice is from women who have been caregivers for their men. It is their hope that the lessons they learned will ease your journey.

- Communicate with your man. You both will be more balanced and able to deal with health-related problems.

- Take time be together without handling, or even thinking about, responsibilities. Be in the moment, watch a movie, or listen to music.

- Learn to let go of your desire to be on top of things. Accept that your daily routines need to change. Adjust your schedule and make it flexible.

- Let friends and family know how they can support both of you. Be specific in your requests for assistance.

- Join a caregivers or disease-related support group.

- Talk with your friends; let your emotions come forth.

- Take care of yourself. Ride a bike, jog, go to the fitness center, take walks, pursue your hobby, write in your journal, or go to lunch with friends. Choose to do what leaves you refreshed.

- Pursue knowledge about your man's disease and the potential treatments. Knowledge will help you to be empowered.

- Tend to your mental, spiritual, and physical needs. That requires your willingness to take time for yourself. It is well worth letting the dishes set in the sink while you do what is good for you.

CHILDREN AS CAREGIVERS

Astonishing At Age Ten

I was in third grade when Mom had breast cancer. As I tell this story, I am a freshman in high school, feeling a bit embarrassed when I recall my reaction to hearing about her diagnosis.

It was a cold, blustery January day in Minnesota. As I trudged up the hill through the snow, I thought, "I bet Mom will have some hot chocolate ready for me."

I opened the front door of our house and bounded inside, very glad to be in the warmth of our home. I tucked my gloves in my coat pocket and hung it on the rack. Then, off with my boots. I ran upstairs, hoping Mom was in the kitchen with a warm drink for me.

I was surprised to find her sitting on the couch with Dad, who was normally at work when I got home from school. They asked what I had done at school that day. I told them about recess, my spelling test, and the neat science project I was working on.

Then Mom said, "Meg, I need to tell you something. Today the doctor told me I have breast cancer."

I said, "Cool."

I still remember the strange expression on Mom's face.

She said, "What?"

She seemed surprised and I sensed that the word "cool" had something to do with her reaction. Now, of course, I understand, but at that point in my life, "cool" was my response to just about everything. It just popped out of my mouth. I couldn't retrieve it and I didn't know what else to say, so I didn't even try to recover.

But I did ask, "Mom, what is breast cancer?"

She said, "It's a disease. Do you know the meaning of the word disease?"

"Yes," I said. I learned about disease in our science class. "I know it makes people sick."

"You're right, Meg," Mom said. "Because of the breast cancer disease, I need to have surgery. I'll be in the hospital for a few days but Dad will be here to take care of you and your brother, Alex."

That seemed okay, as long as she wasn't gone too long.

After she came home, she needed chemotherapy. Alex and I went with Dad to pick her up at the cancer center. We thought it was great because the nurses gave us candy.

One afternoon I said, "Hey, Mom—you get to sit in those neat chairs, watch TV and eat candy. That's cool!"

Oops! There's that word again.

Mom simply said, "This is NOT cool."

I began to think about what I could do to help Mom and others who had breast cancer. I'd heard of walk-a-thons to raise money for charities.

I thought, "That's it. I'll ask my friend, Sharon, if she wants to do a bike-a-thon with me."

We rode our bikes and asked neighbors to support us. They did! With their encouragement and generosity, we raised $250. Mom was so surprised when we showed her the envelope filled with five, ten and twenty dollar bills.

She took us to the *Susan G. Komen Race for the Cure* office where we were greeted by a nice woman who asked, "What can I do for you?"

I handed her the envelope and said, "My mom has breast cancer. I hope this money will help find a way to make her well."

The lady's mouth actually dropped open when she looked into the envelope. She asked, "Where did you get all of this money?"

I told her the story about our bike-a-thon.

I saw tears in her eyes and asked, "Why are you crying?"

She said, "I am deeply touched by what you have done, Meghan."

My mom was beaming with pride as she stood by my side.

She said, "Meg did all this on her own. She asked permission to ride her bike a lot that week but I didn't have any idea that she was on this mission. She surprised me with the money and told me she wanted to help people with breast cancer get well. She knew it was alright to ask friends for contributions because it was for a good cause."

Sharon and I looked at Mom and the *Race for the Cure* woman. We realized we were making a difference in our small world.

Unexpected Publicity

A few days later, a man from a local television station called Mom. He asked if she and her children were willing to be interviewed.

"Yes," she answered.

The TV crew arrived at our home the following morning, which I definitely thought was "cool." They asked me to ride my bike so they could shoot footage (that was a new word for me) of what I did to raise the money to fight breast cancer.

I rode my bike up the block and back home while the cameraman filmed me in action. Then we all went into our living room. Mom and I answered the reporter's questions about the bike-a-thon. My little brother told the reporter about the giggle-jar he made. Although, Alex was only five years old, he conveyed his thoughts and feelings quite clearly.

He said, "Sometimes I feel sad because my mom is sick. But I feel better after I hold this jar to my ear. Every time I do that, I start giggling. And I really like to watch Mom put it by her ear. She starts grinning and then giggles. That makes me happy."

The reporter and cameraman took turns holding Alex's giggle jar to their ears. They started giggling and soon we were all laughing.

After the news team left, Alex and I chattered excitedly about our upcoming TV appearance. At six o'clock p.m. that same day, we were glued to the television set. Wow! There we were, Mom looking beautiful wearing a green bandana to cover her baldhead, and Alex and I enthusiastically telling our stories. We were surprised and happy that they showed so much of our interview. What a thrill.

"It's Only Hair"

Before our television debut, Mom had been strong for us but she wasn't very happy as clumps of hair fell from her head. She bought a wig but only wore it twice. She preferred to wear a hat or put a bandana around her bald head.

One Saturday afternoon, Mom asked, "Meg, is it alright with you if I take off this hat? My head is itching a lot."

"Mom," I said emphatically, "it's only hair!"

From then on she wore head coverings simply by choice, disregarding others' expectations.

Alex and I decided to show Mom our support so we cut off most of our hair. When we walked into the kitchen to surprise Mom, she laughed and hugged us.

"Let's go," she said.

She took us to TCBY for ice cream. Mom's shiny bald head and our heads with tooth-pick short fringe did attract attention as we entered the treat shop. Alex and I felt proud because we were showing support for our mother. If you'll pardon the pun, we were all facing this disease "head-on."

Classroom Trouble Makers

Mom worked at my elementary school. One afternoon she walked into my classroom to give the teacher an envelope. She wore a green bandana, which I thought nothing of until she left. My friend had overheard three boys making mean remarks about Mom's appearance.

She said, "Hey, stop! She has cancer."

They were speechless for a few moments.

Then they turned to me and said, "I'm so sorry. I didn't mean it. I'm really sorry."

I was amazed that the class trouble-makers apologized. I thanked my friend for speaking up. I knew I could count on her for support.

Mom met adversity and won her battle against breast cancer. I admired her and marveled at how well she handled work and home, still giving Alex and I lots of attention and love, while she was undergoing chemotherapy. There was no doubt in my mind that she was an amazing person. She is to this day.

As a Child, Then a Teenager

I was a young girl, unable to comprehend the gravity of what having breast cancer meant to Mom and to our family. In fifth grade, I was learning about geography, math and science. My mind was occupied with school, friends and roller skating. When mom told me she had breast cancer I thought nothing of it. After all, when I came home from school she was there giving me and my younger sister, Gloria, cookies and milk. Life seemed normal to me as the three of us sat at the kitchen table, talking about our days and laughing together. Mom had a great sense of humor and, even though she was sick, managed to do a lot with us.

Mom handled things in a unique way. I remember one of the first things she did after she had a radical mastectomy. The word breast was taboo in conversation at that time, however, when Gloria and I asked, "What is a mastectomy? What does it look like?" she simply removed her blouse and showed us everything.

She took time to explain things and even showed us her imitation breast while she was wearing it. She handled herself well and remained cognizant of our need to know what was happening.

After all of her hair fell out, it became a special event for Gloria and me to go wig shopping with Mom. We had fun. We were allowed to try on long blonde wigs, curly brunette styles, and one that was deep red in color with bangs that fell low on my forehead and covered my eyes. We laughed, and clowned around. We modeled wigs for the store owner who joined right in with the fun. We helped Mom decide on a pretty short, auburn wig that looked totally natural. We thought she was the most beautiful mother in the world.

Mom was an exceptionally strong woman who fought hard to win the battle against breast cancer. She never broke down in front of us but I do remember hearing her cry behind her closed bedroom door. At the time, I did not realize the challenge she faced.

Eventually, Mom had a five year reprieve from cancer. During those few years life was normal in our home. But then the oncologist discovered the cancer had metastasized to other organs in her body. By the time the tumors were discovered, the cancer had spread and she became seriously ill.

As a teenager, I was buying morphine at the pharmacy for my mother, permitted only because the pharmacist knew me. I worked at the drug store. Although I picked up the prescribed pain relievers for her, I was never able to give her the injections. I just couldn't do it. If she was in severe pain and no one else was home to give her the morphine, I called my grandmother, who lived nearby. She immediately appeared at our front door and gave Mom the injection she needed.

I felt the weight of caring for Mom. As a teenager, that was tough! Suddenly, I needed to learn how to do the laundry, clean the house, and prepare dinner. The cooking part was a challenge but I managed.

However, I became extremely rebellious. I did everything possible to avoid being home; but then another part of me kicked into gear. I wanted to help my mother.

I was seventeen years old. I had my driver's license. I drove Mom to her radiation treatments and chemotherapy sessions at the cancer center. I wheeled her to our car, helped her into the front seat, put the wheelchair in the trunk, and drove to the clinic. I was there so often that the nurses all knew me by name and talked with me about my upcoming high school graduation. The staff treated me well but it was hard to see Mom receiving chemo treatments.

During my senior year in high school I took only four classes. I was out of school by noon and was supposed to be going home to take care of Mom. But, I was rebellious and insecure. There were times I chose not to go home until late afternoon. I vividly remember the time I walked through our front door and found Mom struggling to do things alone. That bothered me, especially when she was in severe pain. I tried to be of more help around the house but that was not easy.

My mother was determined to live long enough to see me graduate from high school. On June 19, I walked down the aisle in my cap and gown and reached out to touch Mom as she sat in her wheelchair at the front of the auditorium. She was beaming with pride and I was grateful that she could be at my commencement ceremony.

She Knew

My mother knew when she was going to die. I don't know how, but I am certain she did. Dad had planned to take the four of us to go to the lake in August. The day before we were to leave home, Mom was hospitalized. Dad wanted to cancel the trip but Mom was insistent that he and Gloria go ahead with their plans. However, she wanted me to stay home. I believe she wanted me by her side when she died, two days later.

Unspoken Grief

The entire family was at our house shortly after she passed on. We each handled the loss in our own ways. However, we did share one thing. Every one of us "went internal." We never talked about our grief.

There was not even a funeral or memorial service. To this day, I don't know where Mom's body was placed. Dad didn't tell any of his six children and no one asked. Without having had some type of recognition of her life and death, something to acknowledge her passing, we had no closure. We all had known her death was imminent but I don't think anyone had an inkling of how to deal with it when it actually occurred. It was treated simply as, she was here yesterday; she is gone today. Close that chapter. My family would not open themselves to vulnerability by mentioning how they felt.

For years following Mom's death, I continued to find it difficult for to express my feelings about anything. I had lengthy discussions with a counselor about the anger I carried towards Dad because he prevented our honoring Mom's life and experiencing closure. I have overcome that anger but I still hold my emotions and thoughts close to myself. Although I have grown, I continue to feel the hurt from losing my mother and not having been able to honor her life with some type of recognition by my family.

Teaching Caregiving to a Young Child

My daughter, Karen, taught her son to be a caregiver at a very young age. She was a special education teacher and he loved to go to her school so he could play with the students in her classroom. Before each visit, she reminded him that her students had special needs and may act a little silly or be gruff. One day I took him to Karen's classroom. The girls ran up excitedly and told him they were glad he came to play. However, one of the older boys slugged him hard on the arm.

He calmly looked up at that big boy and said, "You know I'm only six and that hurt."

He had already learned a great deal about understanding others in need.

As my grandson grew older, he knew what it meant to be a caregiver. He volunteered to care for an elderly man and woman, and he organized neighbors to help the couple. They scheduled food deliveries, ran errands, and took turns mowing the lawn or shoveling snow. If the couple needed anything, they simply called one of those on their neighborhood "caregiving committee."

He carried into adulthood the lessons my daughter taught him when he was a little boy. I have heard him tell others that a caregiver lightens the load for someone in need and he is happy to be able to be one of those people.

Words of Wisdom
Children Who Felt the Impact of Disease

"Our entire family felt the impact of my sister's disease. Life changed in our house. Schedules were rearranged, time with my parents was limited, and sometimes I felt neglected."

—William

Children are resilient but, during a crisis, they need an extra dose of support and encouragement. Children, some now adults, shared the following suggestions for kids touched by disease in their families.

- Ask an adult how you can help. Your support is important.

- Draw pictures for your loved one. Ask if he would like you to sing. Your song will brighten their day. However, make sure he is feeling up to a little entertainment.

- If you are feeling sad, talk to your mom, dad, aunt, uncle, your teacher, your youth minister or another adult who understands what is happening in your life.

- It is absolutely okay to talk with your friends. Do so.

- Ask the one who is sick, "How can I help you?"

- Think about what you need versus what you want.

- Talk to your parents. Let them know if you are troubled. Tell them why. Let them help you figure out what to do to make you feel better.

From a Teenager's Perspective

- Take care of yourself. If you need a break, talk with your mom or dad and arrange a time to go out with your friends, go to a movie, hiking, biking, or make time to listen to music or read something you enjoy.

- Ask questions about your loved one's disease. Knowledge lends understanding and you will feel more up to facing the reality of the situation.

- You can express your love and be a major helper by doing the laundry, preparing meals, running errands, and baby-sitting for a younger sibling.

- You may feel an urge to rebel and run away from life at home. However, if you talk to your parents, a school counselor, or another adult you respect, you will probably be able to work out some of your anger and overcome your fears.

- Lack of confidence is likely to make you uptight. If you are taking on new responsibilities, simply ask someone to clarify how to perform those tasks.

CAREGIVING PARENTS

A Mother's Anguish and a Beautiful Gift

Saturday, August 18, 7:30 pm. We had just returned home from a day of sightseeing and were ready to take off our shoes and relax. Not more than five minutes after we walked in the door, the phone rang. It was my daughter, Katie, calling. She chatted for a minute or two, trying to be casual and not to frighten me with the news she was about to share.

Then she said, "Mom, I'm calling for a particular reason tonight. He will be alright but Jack (my son) was injured in a skydiving accident today. He tried to call you collect from a pay phone in the emergency room but you weren't home so he asked me to try to reach you. He is at St. Francis Hospital in Poughkeepsie, New York."

My heart sank. I felt my body trembling as I dialed the number for the emergency room in a hospital a continent away.

A woman answered, "ER."

I said, "I was told I could reach my son, Jack, at this number. He is a patient in…"

She politely interrupted.

She said, "Yes, just a moment."

Time stood still. That few seconds seemed like an hour.

I heard Jack say, "Mom?"

"Yes, Jack—are you alright?" I asked with a lump in my throat. "What happened?"

He said, "I was sky-diving, making my 50th jump. The wind shifted as I neared the ground. I tried to compensate but made a very hard landing. I have a severely fractured sacrum."

"Alright, Jack, I'm on my way. I will call just as soon as I make my airline reservations to let you know when I will be there."

"Thank you Mom, Thank you," he said.

As I returned the phone to its base, my husband appeared right by my side and held me close as I cried.

He asked, "What is it? What happened to Jack?"

I relayed the story to him. He grabbed the news with compassion and helped make plans for me to be on the earliest possible flight to New York.

Sunday morning I departed McCarran Airport. The long flight cross-country seemed like it would never end. When I finally arrived at LaGuardia at 6:30 p.m.,

I rented a car and headed towards Poughkeepsie. The sun set within fifteen minutes. In the dark, driving narrow, curving roads through small towns with few lights, I navigated Highway 9 for three hours. Not knowing just where I was going did not help the stress I already felt. What a relief when I finally spotted the hospital sign.

It was 11:00 pm. I was in a hurry but did not see an accessible door. I spotted a nurse walking towards the employees' entrance. I called to her. She must have seen the tension on my face and heard it in my voice as I asked her to let me go through the door with her. She did so willingly and directed me to the orthopedic unit.

The elevator door opened on the fourth floor. I walked through the quiet hall to the nurses' station. Both night nurses looked up from their work.

I said, "I'm Jack's mom," and immediately thought they must be wondering, "Jack who?"

Not so. They knew Jack and greeted me with warmth.

"Is he sleeping?" I asked.

"Yes," they replied, "but that's ok."

"No", I don't want to wake him," I said.

At that point, both nurses said, compassionately but firmly, "Yes, you do. He told all of us that his mom would be arriving tonight and asked that you please wake him."

I walked into his hospital room, gently touched his shoulder and said, "Jack, its Mom."

His head turned towards me and he smiled.

He said, "Thank you for coming, Mom."

We talked for two hours, which was amazing since he was under the influence of pain medication and I was exhausted from the events of the past twenty-four hours.

I reached my hotel about 1:30 in the morning. I checked in, went to my room, and fell into bed. The following morning, the phone rang. It was Katie.

She said, "Mom. Jack just called. He didn't want to wake you but he is in a lot of pain."

I jumped out of bed, threw on my clothes, and quickly drove the three miles to the hospital. I hurried to his room. I stopped at the doorway where I saw the multi-colored striped curtain pulled around his bed. I heard the physical therapist (PT) talking to Jack.

It was the first time they had met and she was ready to help. She told Jack how she would administer physical therapy but expected him to let her know the level of pain he experienced. She would adjust the treatments accordingly. Jack was willing to try whatever was necessary.

Seconds later, I felt like my gut was torn from my body. Patty, who would come to be his PT angel, had put her hand behind his back and asked him to try to raise himself. The intense, excruciating pain caused an involuntary, primal scream to come from the very depths of his being.

I stood in the hallway, only four feet from Jack. I needed to stay out of the way while Patty helped him but my heart ached and I honestly shared some of his physical pain.

Compassionate, knowledgeable, PT Patty was Jack's physical therapist for the next ten days. She was an angel of compassion and understanding with a great deal of ability to analyze his situation and develop a flexible treatment plan. Jack received pain medication as needed and received physical therapy twice a day. PT Patty provided both of us with instructions on how to continue his therapy when she was not available.

She told us, "Jack's injury is serious. He has numerous fractures in the sacrum that causes excruciating pain because all of the body's nerves and muscles join in the sacrum."

He tried everything she asked of him. She was so attuned to his pain that she would slowly try one movement and then another. She taught me how to adjust the bed, lift his legs, and help him exercise.

I spent the days and evenings with Jack. We talked. When he felt he could rest, I read a book, walked outside, or went shopping for a few things he needed. About midweek, he insisted I go somewhere to have a nice lunch.

Sitting on an outdoor deck of a small restaurant, overlooking the river, I watched tugboats pass by while children played in a lovely small park. Taking those couple of hours to rejuvenate was what I needed. Caregivers do need time to renew their own strength.

Jack was not mobile but he worked via telephone and through his laptop, staying connected with his co-workers in New York City. Aunts, uncles and friends called. An outpouring of love and concern came from near and far.

His dad and sister lived in Colorado. It was exceedingly difficult for them to be so many miles away but Jack and I talked with them several times a day, filling them in on his status and prognosis. Jack's dad planned to fly to New York a day or two before Jack was released from the hospital, so he could learn what he could do to adapt Jack's apartment to his limited mobility, and, of course, drive him back to the city. He planned to stay until Jack was well situated.

Meanwhile, Katie was helping from a long distance position. She provided mental relief for Jack when she volunteered to handle the automobile situation. He had rented a car in New York City and drove to the skydiving "Ranch" in Gardner. The vehicle was still setting there. She contacted Avis Car Rental, arranged for them to pick up the car, and took care of all the details.

While all of this was happening, my husband was still at our home in Nevada. He was also experiencing the helplessness of being so far away, and was concerned about Jack and about me. We talked nightly. I didn't know how long I would be in Poughkeepsie but he still, even though he said he missed me greatly, supported my staying as long as necessary. He listened to what was happening at my end of the telephone line and shared what was happening in his world.

Jack made great progress. He slowly moved from being able to sit on the side of the bed, which was a huge achievement, to putting his weight on his feet, then sitting in a wheel chair, and gradually taking a few steps with a walker. Suddenly, he seemed to have made miraculous improvement. PT Patty was proud of him and we were elated when the doctor said he was ready to move from the orthopedic unit to the physical rehabilitation unit the following day. Dr. Samson anticipated he would be released from the hospital within the week.

Day 10. I walked into his new room—rehab! Out of hospital gowns and into his own clothing. Therapy would prepare Jack to be able to care for himself at home.

That was all good news but I was there to say farewell. He needed to be on his own and I needed to be home. We chatted a bit and then he told me he had experienced a setback during the night.

He said, "Mom, I'm so glad you told me that I may have a set back after all the progress I made yesterday. I did last night. The pain was intense when I tried to sit on the edge of the bed. It hurt like hell. That depressed me, but then I remembered what you had said. I thought about your reminder again this morning when I experienced agonizing pain; I realized it was just a setback. I knew things would improve. I'm so glad you told me not to be surprised if that happened, Mom."

He was feeling better and expected to make significant progress in the physical rehab unit. There was an excellent medical staff to help him heal. He felt more confident about his recovery, as did I.

It was time for me to leave. Our farewells have always had a touch of sadness knowing we wouldn't see each other again for a while but this one was more poignant than most. He told me how much he appreciated what I had done for him. He had already thanked me and expressed his gratitude innumerable times, but he said it once again. I told him that I was honored that he wanted me to be with him through this traumatic ordeal.

We hugged, exchanged an emotional mother son moment as we looked into one another's eyes, and tried to smile as we said good-bye.

Jack said, "Don't worry, Mom. I'll be fine."

I answered, "I know. I'll talk to you tomorrow."

A nurse interrupted our farewell but we still said, "I love you" to each other.

On the flight home, tears brimmed on the edge of my eyes. I blinked them back. The next day, at home, I cried. I felt relief for Jack's positive prognosis, pain for what he had encountered, and grateful that from this tragic accident I received a gift I treasure dearly—our mother-son bond was strengthened with super glue.

Just Thirteen Years Old

Her soccer coach said, "Carol, if we were down by five and only had two minutes to play, you are the one I would put in the game."

His words succinctly described my teen-age daughter's personality. She had an athlete's persistence, a drive to win. She loved to play soccer and basketball. Suddenly her life changed, as did mine.

Carol had been having headaches. She was very tired but when she lay down to rest the pain in her head became more intense. Then she began vomiting frequently.

I called our pediatrician who, fortunately, was willing to take time late Friday afternoon to be exceptionally thorough in analyzing her condition.

After asking Carol for detailed answers to a number of questions, he turned to me and said, "You need to go to Children's Hospital right now."

I said, "What do you mean right now? I need to call my husband, make arrangements for someone to care for our other children…" I thought, "This just wasn't in the plan today."

Dr. Sam said, "You must go now!"

That was the first lesson I learned in this unfolding chapter of our lives. My flexibility would be essential in the days to come. I drove straight to the hospital. The health care team met us and zipped Carol off to perform tests. I became frightened and called my husband.

"Tom," I said, "please come to the hospital. Something is terribly wrong and I can't do this alone. The doctors have only told me that they've called in specialists."

He arrived just as one of the physicians, Dr. Tim, was telling me that Carol had brain cancer. My heart raced. My stomach felt as though it had been hit with a baseball bat.

I thought, "But my daughter just became a teenager. She's only thirteen years old. How can she have cancer?"

The oncologist interrupted my thoughts when he walked into the family waiting room and said, "Dr. Tim is right. You don't have a lot of time to think about this. We need to do something quickly. If we wait, Carol could suffer permanent brain damage. She can wait only until tomorrow morning."

Tom and I stayed with Carol in her hospital room that night. Suddenly, she had double vision. She asked more questions. I wasn't yet ready to tell her she had cancer but I did explain that she had hydrocephalus. I told her the surgeon would insert a shunt that would act like a drain and relieve the pressure on her brain. She did not seem overly concerned about the procedure. She just wanted relief from her headaches.

I don't think she and I slept more than thirty minutes that night but Tom was sound asleep in a chair in the corner of the room.

Carol, with her dry wit, said, "Isn't it comforting to know that Dad is here and he will be well rested in the morning? Reliable, trustworthy, loyal…and rested."

We both laughed.

It seemed to be an exceptionally long night but the sun finally rose. Dr. Robert explained to Carol that she had brain cancer and needed surgery immediately. At the vulnerable age of thirteen, my daughter understood what was happening. She knew the disease could cause death.

She said, "I don't want to die, Mom. I don't know if I will, but if I do, it won't be so scary because I know Jesus will be there."

She said things like that every once in a while, which I considered a positive thing. It made me feel better to know that she would be at peace if she did pass on.

But there were many times when I simply cried out, "Please God, no!"

Following surgery, Carol was given a protocol developed specifically for children having the same rare type of cancer. Physicians throughout the world worked together to find a cure for these young people. Fifteen years ago, Carol would have had four months to live but now, due to amazing medical progress, she had a great chance of moving on with her life at a normal rate.

What's normal? I guess that's all relative but we looked forward to watching her run down the soccer field again and to cheering her on as she shot hoops on the basketball court.

After six weeks of simultaneous chemotherapy and radiation, Carol was given the gift of six weeks without treatment. During that hiatus, sparkle returned to her eyes and she was more energetic than she had been for a long time. We celebrated all road signs that pointed toward recovery.

I Became My Daughter's Nurse

Carol resumed chemo treatment for another six months. During the first month we spent two days per week in the hospital. She did so well that we were able to implement a home plan and I became her nurse. My responsibilities included giving her intravenous (IV) chemotherapy for the next five months. The best part of this new approach was that she was home.

Financial Challenges

As a child's caregiver, I was in an unstable financial position. Carol was disabled but I was not; I wasn't eligible for financial assistance even though I needed to quit my job to care for Carol. I wanted to work part-time but that was not an option at the company where I was employed. I had no choice but to resign.

I needed to be home for my daughter for more reasons than administering and monitoring IVs. I was on call for Carol. She had returned to classes on a part-time basis. When she was tired, she called me. Without delay, I drove to school and brought her home. When I received her calls I knew she had pushed as long as she could that day and needed complete rest. Typical of Carol, those were times exemplary of her athlete's persistence tempered with her player's understanding of her own body.

She said, "Mom, when I need to give one-hundred fifty percent in a game, I can do that. But I also know when I need to slow down to conserve energy for the next big thrust that may be required again."

I also wanted to be home with Carol to put my arms around her when she was feeling so poorly that she just wanted to be held, to prepare foods that wouldn't make her nauseous, and do whatever I could to ease her suffering when the after-effects of chemo took its toll on her body.

Caring for Carol was indeed an honor, especially since she was a teenager, and yet allowed me to share in what may be the worst moments of her life. I was grateful to be able to be with her during such a difficult time.

My Sons Needed Me Too

While Carol received the lion's share of my attention during her treatment and recovery, my sons still wanted and needed my love, support, and physical care. They needed their mother, especially when things seemed to be out of balance.

They were younger than Carol and grew up faster than many boys their ages as we all moved through this difficult time in our lives. They learned to ask for what they needed. We spent a lot of time discussing and clarifying whether they wanted or needed something. They shared their feelings and let me know that they needed personal attention each day.

I tried to heed their verbal and nonverbal messages as we moved forward. I took time to answer their questions about Carol's disease and how we could help her to get better. I was aware of their developmental levels and gave them information accordingly. I didn't want to overwhelm them with a lot of explanations and reasoning that they couldn't assimilate.

They certainly had their ups and downs, as did all of us. There were times they were just plain angry that this had happened to Carol and to them. They were angry with God, Carol, and me.

There was more than one instance when I overheard one brother tell the other, "I hate this!" and immediately saw them head to their sister's room to ask if there was anything they could do for her. I allowed their emotional outbursts but I also opened my arms and heart to them.

One time I had spent five minutes with Carol but my son was sure I had been with her at least an hour. That was a warning sign! He needed my attention. I took him to dinner at Perkins, one of his favorite things to do. Being aware of those signals and following up by giving attention and one-on-one time eased their frustration. I learned to refill their P.U.s (personal units), as my friend referred to kids' needs.

Our Marriage Felt the Pressure

Tom also needed my attention. Our stress level was off the charts. We knew about the enormous divorce rate of parents with children who have chronic illnesses. The situation and demands placed a huge strain on a marriage. We worked to stay connected.

I vividly recall the time I had a true awakening.

I thought, "Well God, now I know why you had me marry this man. He has such strength and unbelievable faith. Anytime I need him, he's there. He is a man of few but very wise words. His faith and wisdom were apparent when Carol's second brain tumor was discovered.

The oncologist said, "With one tumor like Carol has on her brain, the survival rate is sixty percent. But with this additional tumor, the survival rate is only thirty percent."

I cried out, "No! Carol's going to die!"

Tom said, "Die? What do you mean die? I heard she has a thirty percent chance to live."

"Oh, Honey," I said to him, "you are absolutely right. What am I thinking?"

From that moment on, we considered medical statistics as only information to be considered. We knew Carol was an individual person, not a number. We had a great deal of faith in our medical team and those doctors agreed with us on our perspective of statistics. We altered our thinking and accepted the challenges that laid before us.

After much discussion, Tom and I agreed that if Carol decided to let go of her battle against cancer we would understand that she was ready to be with God. We would tell her that we understand, we love her, and would be by her side to help her gracefully move through transition from this life to one with Jesus.

However, What to Tell Carol?

After Tom and I talked, I went to see Carol in the infusion room where she was receiving a chemo drip through an IV. I didn't want her to see me looking as though I had been crying for an hour, but I had. I slowly walked down the hall, wondering what I would say to my precious daughter. Once again, I was aware of her developmental stage.

"I don't think she's ready for those frightening statistics," I thought. "But what will I say?"

The words came naturally once I was with her.

I said, "Carol, when you were diagnosed with asthma I was concerned for you. Now you've been diagnosed with cancer and I am concerned for you."

I intentionally avoided the word frightened. I thought that may scare her.

I said, "When you have trouble with anything, I'm concerned. That's a 'mom thing.' You need to let me have my 'mom stuff' which is different from what you need."

She agreed and we talked about the steps she would take. I appreciated truly open communication with my daughter, family and the medical team. Perhaps more importantly, I realized that if I allowed myself to receive help from the spirit within, I could easily find answers.

Outpouring of Support

I still thank God, my family and friends for being there for us through this ordeal. People amazed us with their generous acts of kindness. Neighbors and friends ran errands for us, brought meals, had Carol's brothers over to their homes, and were on-call to do whatever was needed. Carol's teachers were compassionate and understood her situation. They worked with her so she wouldn't fall far behind in her school work. The nurses on the children's oncology unit gave parents relief and support when it was most needed. Carol's school friends and many dear people in our lives sent cards, stopped by our house to see her, and called frequently.

Our neighbors were amazing. Through their all-out efforts, they raised $25,000 for what they dubbed *The Carol Fund*. The story of the incredible walkathon, *Our Community Walked for Carol*, can be found in Chapter Nine.

Friends Want to Know

We received an amazing number of e-mails and phone calls from friends and family asking about Carol's condition and wanting to know how they could help. I created a website to provide that information in an easily accessible format. Creating and updating the website also acted as a release valve for me, much like journaling is for many people experiencing trying times.

As a caregiver, you may want to create your own website to stay in touch with others while your time is consumed with caring for your loved one. It is a valuable tool for staying in touch with friends and family. Remember, they truly want to be of service and through your website, you are able to let them know how they can support you and your family. (Additional information about the website can be found as *Carol's Website* in Chapter Four, *Communication*.)

Survivor

Carol is a survivor in many ways. She triumphed over brain cancer and is playing soccer and basketball again. She is back in school and loving life. She will soon be fourteen years old, chronologically. She is about eighty years old in wisdom and is an inspiration to many.

Our family faced obstacles and bolted over barriers. We came out on the other side very connected, much like a closely knit sweater with colors of individualism and the loving warmth of alpaca wool. I thank God. I thank the innumerable people who provided us support and love.

I Was A "Fixer"

I tried to be constantly positive while I cared for my daughter, Karen, during her treatments for cancer. When Karen had cancer the first time, I had to come to grips with reality. I had to accept that I could not change her physical condition.

All my life I had been what I called a "fixer." I had always been able to make things better until disease raised its ugly head. Suddenly, I was up against something in my life that I could not mend. I realized that putting my requirements to make everything better was not helping anyone, certainly not Karen. When I finally allowed myself to accept the circumstances and simply be there to support and love Karen, a huge burden was lifted from my shoulders.

Before that epiphany, I had worked myself into a mental frenzy. As a parent, I felt helpless. I knew I could not reverse what had happened to Karen.

As I drove home from work one afternoon, a police officer stopped me. At that point, I realized I did not have any idea where I was, geographically speaking. I had been driving in a mental fog, preoccupied with Karen and all that her situation encompassed.

The officer walked towards my car. I rolled down the window and heard him ask, "Are you alright?"

I said, "Yes, I am. Why do you ask?"

He said, "I have been following you for seven miles and you are driving somewhat erratically, as though you were the only one on the road."

"I'm so sorry, Officer," I said. My daughter is having her third surgery for cancer tomorrow and all of my thoughts are with her."

He did not give me a ticket. Instead, he asked if I wanted him to follow me home to be sure I arrived safely.

I said, "No, it's not much further. I will be alright. Thank you for bringing me back to reality."

That police officer may have been an angel who prevented a serious accident because he snapped me out of the mental and emotional fog that surrounded me.

After that, I was able to focus on what Karen needed rather than what I thought I could fix for her. I do still carry one fear; fear of losing my daughter. It seemed that each time she had a medical appointment, another problem surfaced. I remained calm as she told me about the latest developments, but after I hung up the phone, I sat down and cried. My heart was breaking. My tears became sobs of despair.

I felt relief when I recalled what a good child she had been and that, as a teenager, she did not get into trouble; but she was constantly seeking fun. She wanted to have a good time, to party, and do whatever she found enjoyable. Now I am so thankful that she lived life to its fullest during her teen years because she will never again be able to be so free and physically active. Those capabilities were cut short, abruptly.

I learned an important lesson: the most important thing a caregiver can do is to let go of menial tasks and focus on moments with their loved one. I treasure the times Karen and I have shared, and pray we will have many more years together.

Teen Years + Chemotherapy = Rebellion

At the time, little did I know that Ken and I would both become cancer survivors. I just knew that my teenage son, Ken, was diagnosed with cancer, and I was deeply shaken.

The physician at University Hospital examined the lump on my son's neck.

It was obvious that Ken's condition was critical when the doctor said, "Ken, I want you to spend the night here and we'll begin treatment in the morning."

I said, "Of course, we'll stay."

In retrospect, I realized that speaking for Ken was a mistake. I knew this was serious, but Ken had his own independent thoughts.

He said, "No, Mom. I don't want to stay. I want to see my friends."

Hearing that was difficult because I didn't know what was going through his mind. I couldn't help but wonder if he thought he was going to die.

I respected his wishes and said, "Alright."

We drove home with very few words being spoken. Ken wasn't ready to talk. He and his buddies went out and he didn't return home until two o'clock in the morning. I had very little sleep that night.

By six a.m., we were in the car driving to the hospital. The oncologist was waiting for us and introduced us to others who would be on Ken's medical team. He told me that Ken would be treated for stage-four cancer.

Stage four! I was terribly frightened.

The medical team was ready. They immediately began to administer chemotherapy, which included five drugs. I thought that seemed like a lethal dose. After every single treatment, Ken vomited. Watching my sixteen-year old son go through all of that agony was the hardest thing I have ever done.

"Please let me be the one, not Ken," I thought. Over and over I questioned, "Why does he have to go through this? To make him stronger? He's strong enough now."

I realized the pain I was bearing would not help Ken. I decided to be strong for him and muster all the support I could garner. I didn't yet know the obstacles that lay ahead.

Just being a teenager can be difficult in itself but those raging hormones combined with the heavy doses of chemotherapy struck a note of rebellion in Ken. Maybe "note" is an understatement. There were days he absolutely refused to go for treatment.

On a couple of occasions he yelled at me, "I'm not going to let anybody put that poison in my body!"

"What could I do?" I asked myself.

It was impossible for me to pick him up and put him in the car. I knew he had already learned to make decisions for himself, but my worry was intense. I was certain he knew what needed to be done; however, I also knew it would be done when he decided it was time. I had seen that in Ken before.

It was difficult to communicate with my son during his treatment period. For instance, we began conversations in normal tones of voice, only to have them escalate into shouting matches. Other times it was the opposite; we bellowed at one another and then settled into a rational, calm conversation.

We have had a rough relationship at times, and I have always thought of Ken as my challenging child.

I asked myself, "What's different now?" I answered my own question. "We may be making life and death decisions," I thought.

I was scared.

Ken endured suffering and won the battle against his disease. I don't know if I could have done as well when I was sixteen. At the age of twenty, he had regained fifteen pounds and his blood count was excellent. It took about two and a half years to recover from his treatment.

I asked him to walk the survivor circuit with me at the *American Cancer Society Relay for Life*. He agreed.

As we made our way around the relay track, we paused. I looked into my son's eyes and said, "Ken, you are my hero. You are the reason I was able to make it through my personal battle with cancer."

He smiled and put his arm around my shoulders. We walked on.

An Interview with Team K

I met "Team K" at the *Relay for Life*, a fund raising event sponsored by the *American Cancer Society*. Jerry's and Betty's two children, Keith and Suzie, were with them. Keith, only five years old, had leukemia. He had been in and out of hospitals receiving treatment since his second birthday. His sister, Suzie, was in eighth grade and a strong supporter of her little brother.

During our conversation, they agreed to be interviewed for this book so they could share their story with families who might learn from their experience.

Suzie: Our family referred to ourselves as "Team K," meaning Keith's team. We pulled together as one strong force to help Keith face the challenges of getting well.

Jerry: Keith has been on a steroid called Dexamethasone. As he continued to grow, the drug seemed to have a more intense impact on his behavior. Within twenty minutes of being given the steroid, the effect was quite obvious. For instance, if I handed him a toy truck and he did not want it, he would blame me for handing it to him wrong. He would carry on like that for the full five days he received Dextamethasone. It was clear to us that when that dosage was completed, he resumed being his normal, delightful self until the next round. It was very difficult for him and for all of us.

He also experienced sleeping disorders and was hungry throughout the five days. He even chewed his shirt, as though he was teething. I do not think his teeth actually hurt but they must have felt strange. The steroids weakened his bone structure and prevented calcium from entering his bones. He also took 6MP/Methotrexate, which destroyed tooth enamel. His reactions were among the things we didn't expect when we began this journey.

The same was true regarding medical insurance. I thought my family was covered by a good health plan until we were in this situation with Keith. For instance, each time we went to a health care provider the intake person would question us as though we were lying.

I kept asking myself, "Why can't they get this? Why can't someone enter a red flag in their computer that says this child has leukemia?"

Medical expenses were a major concern and it was very difficult to pay the bills until aid was provided. I do consider our family fortunate in one regard, namely, Keith's oncologist. Dr. R told Betty and I that if we could not afford to pay, we should not stop coming. He said he would work something out.

Peg (interviewer): Jerry, please tell me about Keith's disease.

Jerry: Keith's type of leukemia has a seventy percent cure rate with the expectation that five years later, the diseased child will be cancer free. Twenty-five percent of those children may have a relapse, which is a difficult thing to overcome because their young bodies have already taken about all they can endure. Looking at the numbers, some people consider those good odds but if your child is in that twenty-five percent group, it is perplexing and hard to accept.

People didn't always understand what our family went through. They did not know that it was important to us for them to share a little of their time talking and listening. We needed emotional support. Our lives changed drastically.

Betty: Living with this has certainly changed my perspective on many things. One such change I'd like to tell you about is my going to church. With leukemia in our lives, even prayers sounded different to me, and the words in the hymns came to life. Someone in this situation doesn't talk with God about wanting a new car or asking for His help with a small problem. Life is different when a life threatening or serious disease is in your midst. I prayed, "Son of God, please heal my son." Then I needed to prepare myself to accept and deal with whatever happened next.

Peg: Did you also have other sources of strength and support, Betty?

Betty: Yes. Friends and family were supportive. But I was amazed by a strange thing that happened to me. I've discovered that I've become a support person for others. Let me tell you a story.

I was talking with a co-worker whose sister had recently died of cancer. I knew he had not been able to talk with anyone about his loss. I listened and asked questions to help him sort out things in his mind.

When it was time for both of us to get back to our work, he said, "Wow. You have such a strong positive attitude."

At that moment, I realized what a great lesson I had learned from Keith. My little boy never gave up. While in the hospital, his port became infected. As a result, his hand was completely wrapped in bandages. Even though he couldn't use one hand, he wanted to be in the play room with the other young patients. That wrapped hand did not interfere with his determination. He simply used the other hand to pick up the toys. His actions demonstrated to me that if something is important, there are absolutely no boundaries that can't be worked around."

Jerry: You can learn a lot from children.

Betty: And you learn a lot every single day. One important lesson I quickly learned was that I could, and did, enjoy each new day. Even if things didn't go as I liked, I still loved life. And I always reminded myself that I have today!

Jerry: Keith seemed to give us appreciative messages often. His first hospital stay was for three weeks.

When we left the hospital to take him home, he looked at me and exclaimed, "Dad! Look at that. The sky is blue! Look at the green grass and that big tree. Isn't that a pretty tree?"

I have walked by that tree many times and barely noticed it, but Keith saw its beauty, ran up to the tree and gave it a hug. I was looking at the big picture, thinking we may not win this fight.

But Keith's positive attitude was obvious when he said excitedly, "Look at that! Isn't that great?!"

Another time I was mowing the lawn. I've mowed thousands of yards but this time was different. I had to stop the lawn mower four times, once for a dandelion because it was a flower to be saved, twice for lady bugs because Keith didn't want me to run over them, and again for a roly-poly grey bug."

Betty: You should have seen the lawn. His usual straight geometric patterns in the grass looked like a zigzagged maze.

Peg: It appears that you received a lot of strength from Keith. How did you take care of yourselves?

Jerry: I rode my bicycle. For me, that was extremely therapeutic. As I pedaled along the trails or streets I found I was able to let go of my cares. I regained strength during those periods of respite.

I knew several people who had diabetes and I wanted to be an active part of those who were helping to fight that disease. So Suzie and I registered for the thirty-six mile diabetes ride. Keith was diagnosed with leukemia three days prior to the event. You can imagine how I felt. I did not think riding a bicycle was what I wanted to do. But my family and friends insisted that we take that ride. So we did.

As Suzie and I rode through the streets, I was careful to keep both of us to the right. My role as dad had me looking after my thirteen-year-old daughter. We had not trained for the hills we encountered on this ride so by the time we reached the first pit stop, Suzie was exhausted. She decided to stop. The crew provided her transportation back to the starting point.

With gusto, I resumed riding. I felt like I was flying as I pedaled my bicycle at twenty miles per hour. The warm sun, clear skies, and the wind in my face, refreshed me. I was aware that I was alive and I felt wonderful. Much to my surprise, I actually forgot that Keith was in the hospital, facing a potentially life threatening situation. For the better part of six hours I didn't think about what we were facing. I was more concerned about life and what was happening around me as I zipped along the road. That was outstanding therapy! I was strengthened to face our family reality when I returned home.

Bicycling and work were my salvation. My job required my full attention. For eight hours a day my focus was on my work. That was another bit of therapy for me.

The men I worked with were very supportive. One of my coworkers lost a friend to cancer. He understood my feelings and fears. We talked about the disease and the impact it has on family and friends. We seemed to connect and were able to talk on a personal level.

Talking about what was happening to Keith was most helpful. I appreciated the men's support group that was a segment of the Candle Lighters, an organization of parents and others who care for children with leukemia.

Betty: I found a lack of women's support groups. I knew I needed reinforcement but didn't know where to turn. My daughter, Mom, and I pulled together and became very close but I needed to reach outside the family. I heard about an adult cancer support group and decided to sit in on a few of their meetings. Several of the members did not understand why I would want to join them if I was the mother of a child with leukemia. I told them that my son had a life threatening disease and I needed support to remain strong for him. I wanted to learn all I could about helping him. I found, as did the group members, that Keith shared many of the same problems as adult victims of cancer.

One side effect of treatment was restlessness or little sleep. My friends, as they quickly became, from the support group found that to be a common problem. I became creative to find solutions or at least relief in certain situations. Concerning sleep, I suggested turning on the TV and letting cartoons run all night. Not only my young son, but even the adults liked that idea. The support group helped me and, to my surprise, I helped them.

When I returned to those meetings for reunions, I was honored when a man walked up to me and said, "That poem you read at one of our meetings helped me. Thank you."

Others made a point of telling me about how something I had shared helped them in their lives. Their gratitude showed me I made a difference. I was grateful for that beautiful gift.

There is a strong need for people to come together, to learn from one another and perhaps most importantly, to know they can share their feelings, tears, and laughter. The bond and energy created by people in a caring group is incredible.

Peg: You mentioned that as you traveled this road, you encountered unexpected changes in your lives. Would you tell me more about that experience?

Jerry: Yes, there were several. We were not prepared for the medical expenses incurred. We sold land we were close to owning outright. We learned to function with one car rather than two. We changed our work schedules so one of us could be with Keith around the clock; he required special care. Those were a few of the alterations in our daily lives.

My outlook about leukemia turned 180 degrees. Initially, I was afraid and did not have much hope that Keith would overcome his cancer. Three or four months after his diagnosis, I woke up and realized that I did not bring a son in this world to lose him at such a young age. I decided to fight! The oncologist was on our side. He believed we could win. So we marched on. As we moved through our journey, Keith had difficult periods, particularly with some of the treatments he received. As parents, Betty and I felt his pain. We tried everything to alleviate his suffering.

Those who thought we were spoiling him criticized us but we continued to do what we thought was best for him. I happened to speak with an executive from an international toy company who said he almost lost his son to cancer. He spoke of the numerous toys they gave him with the hope that he would think about the gifts that lay ahead rather than the suffering he endured. Some people might believe that parents spoil their sick child, but when you are the mother or father, you will do everything possible to brighten your child's day.

Peg: How did Suzie handle all of this?

Betty: Our daughter, Suzie, was in fifth grade when Keith was diagnosed with leukemia.

We were stunned one evening at home when she blurted out, "I wish I was Keith. He gets everything."

That was a cry for attention. The American Cancer Society gave me a book titled, *Your Sibling Has Cancer.* Suzie wouldn't read the book so I suggested we read it together. Most importantly, it provided an avenue for conversation about her feelings.

During one of those discussions, Suzie asked, "Mom, do you mean that he didn't get sick because I wouldn't let him watch my television?'"

Larry: Guilt. A child life specialist told us that children sometimes feel that way.

She relayed the story of a girl who, in a fit of anger, yelled to her brother, "I wish you were dead."

Two hours later the young boy fell into a swimming pool and drowned. The girl genuinely believed it happened because she wished him dead. It is important to get through to any of those misleading feelings and put them on the table. By addressing those issues, they can be alleviated and the child can understand the reality of what has happened rather than the fantasy they create for themselves.

Peg: Suzie, please tell me what you were thinking and feeling.

Suzie: My uncle died from cancer when I was in third grade. We were very close. I used to call him and talk for hours. He was patient with my childhood questions and continued to answer and discuss topics until I was satisfied. How I enjoyed those conversations! And I know he was pleased to be able to share his experiences and knowledge. I was devastated when cancer took his life. When I was told that Keith had cancer, I was very afraid that he would die too. I will say what helped me was being able to talk with my family.

Peg: When someone is diagnosed with a serious disease, tension in a family can become overwhelming. What do you and Betty do to nourish your family relationships and enhance communication?.

Larry: Our time together was limited, but we used beepers and cell phones to stay connected. (Refer to *Family Connections* in the *Communication* chapter.) We used codes that conveyed 'I need to talk' or 'I made it to work safely.' We made time for each other and for Suzie. Keith received a lot of attention but we always remembered that there were four of us in this family, all with unique needs. We tried to meet those needs.

Betty's brother and mother were great support for us. When our car broke down, they were right there to drive us to wherever we needed to be. They stayed in the hospital with Keith so we could take a break. When Suzie wanted to talk, she did not hesitate to pick up the phone and call Grandma. We were fortunate to have a wonderful support system.

Betty: We are grateful for the support we received from family, friends, co-workers, acquaintances, and the people in our support groups.

Words of Wisdom
Parents Caring for Their Child

"It was heart wrenching to watch our child suffer. We prayed for strength, leaned on one another, and did all we could for our son while he was in treatment for cancer. The rest of our family still needed us—we heeded their call. We were tired. We asked for help—it was there."

—Caregiving Parents

The following advice is from parents who have experienced similar ordeals. They provided suggestions on facing the challenges of a child's disease and continuing to care for the rest of their family.

- Ask health care professionals what to expect in the way of physical and behavioral changes your child may experience while undergoing treatment.

- Help your child find ways to occupy his mind. Play games with him, give him toys and books to divert his attention from suffering, play music, comfort him through touch and hugs, and listen when he wants to talk.

- Let his questions be your guide as to the type of medical information you share with him, keeping in mind his developmental level.

- Take care of yourself. Crying may purge your blues; let it happen and then move on with a brighter outlook toward each day.

Siblings

- Brothers and sisters may be jealous because their sibling is receiving so much attention. Take time for each of your children. Do "normal" activities with them.

- Discuss the situation. Explain the disease.

- Let them know how they can help. Praise their acts of kindness.

- If your child is not asking questions, or seems withdrawn, initiate conversation. He may be carrying a lot of stress or feeling he somehow contributed to his brother's illness. Be aware that children often create their own unfounded guilt.

- Be aware of nonverbal messages they send. A sudden outburst may be a cry for attention.

- Expect outbursts of emotion and, when they occur, remain calm. Give him or her the opportunity to tell you how they are feeling.

Teens with Disease

- Respect your teenager's thoughts and wishes. It may help to recall that stage in your life when you needed to affirm individuality and self-confidence.

- Allow her to make educated decisions about her care.

- Teen years often equate to mood swings. Disease accents their emotions. Be patient.

- Communication with your teen may be difficult. Try to control your tone of voice; avoid shouting matches. Escalating volume just exacerbates the tension.

- Keep in mind that your son or daughter is suffering with mental anguish, as well as physical pain.

- There may be times you feel like you are biting your tongue so you don't explode in front of your teen. Take a deep breath. Then call a friend and vent.

Take Care of Yourself

- Allow flexibility in your own schedule.

- Ask friends to care for your other children occasionally.

- Make a date with your spouse, significant other, or friends. Go out and have a good time.

- Let others help you. It is a gift for them to be able to do something for you and your family.

REVERSED ROLES: ADULT CHILDREN CARE FOR THEIR PARENTS

She Kept Quiet

My mother had been cancer free for fifteen years when suddenly our world turned upside down. Mom's CAT scan revealed a suspicious spot on her left lung. Our family was horribly fearful that her original breast cancer had metastasized; however, the doctor did not think that was the case. But nothing was definite. Even after she had undergone treatment and was doing well we still moved from day to day with trepidation.

I was eleven years old when Mom had cancer the first time. She cared for me and my thirteen year old brother, Ron. She and Dad did all they could to keep "their secret" from us. Ron and I were aware that something was awry, although we didn't understand the full implications of what was happening. We knew Mom had been in the hospital, had a mastectomy, and received chemotherapy treatment. But our young minds didn't comprehend the magnitude of the burden our parents were bearing. Mother never explained her condition to us. She did all she could to allow our innocence of childhood beliefs exist. We thought life was normal.

As an adult, I realized what she must have endured fifteen years earlier. I recalled the times she cried in her bedroom, but always emerged secretly drying her tears, to put dinner on the table or check to be sure we were doing our home-work.

When I became a young woman I heard stories of people with breast cancer. That's when reality hit me. The jolt was strong, leaving me shaken like the time a deer jumped into the road in front of my brake-screeching car.

I trembled as I thought, "Good grief, my mom had breast cancer. She must have gone through a lot of pain. She may have died."

At that point, I had a strong need to talk about it with Mom but she was not ready to have that discussion. I did not like her keeping a secret of something so important.

I lived with this cancer thing for as long as I can remember. The more know-ledge I gained the better I handled certain aspects of the situation. It never became easy. I continued to fear that I could suddenly lose my mother.

While home from college one summer, I took Mom to the clinic for a day-long chemo treatment. That day I gained first-hand knowledge of the intense pain a caregiver feels while watching a loved one undergo treatment. I felt so helpless.

Fifteen years following her double mastectomy, Mom developed lympho-dema. Her arm swelled, likely caused by radiation since the toxins in her lymph nodes accumulated in her arm. She had a lot of discomfort. If she wore a blouse or sweater that was the least bit snug on her upper arm, she felt pain.

One of the greatest memories I have is of Mom and I vacationing together in the Caribbean. She was relaxed and enjoying herself as we sat by the swimming pool bar. I was delighted that she had been willing to put on her bathing suit. She had a towel draped over her swollen arm.

I said, "Mom, why don't you get in the water? No one is watching you. Look around and you'll see that not a single person is even aware of our presence. And why would we care anyway? We're in the islands on vacation!"

She surprised me with her quick response.

She said, "Okay. Here's what I'll do. I'll stand up and then, as you pull my towel away, I'll duck into the water."

I was ecstatic! At last, Mom let go of some of her inhibitions. She allowed her-self to have fun. I think I was happier than Mom was at that moment. My heart went out to her.

Years after that glorious vacation, I received a long distance call from my brother.

He said, "Sis, we have a serious problem."

"What is it?" I asked.

His reply sent a shockwave through me.

"Mom just called and said she wants me to come home this weekend to help her get things together because she's dying of cancer."

"What are you talking about?" I asked.

"I don't know what's going on," he said. "I don't know exactly what's happening but she wants me to help get her papers straightened out. She's sure she has cancer and does not want me to tell you or Dad."

"There it is again," I thought. "Cancer secrecy. She has not even told Dad."

After Ron and I talked, I immediately called Mom. Needless to say, she quickly realized that Ron had told me her secret and she was not happy about that.

After she calmed down, she said, "I have cancer and I remember what I went through fifteen years ago. I am <u>not</u> going for treatment. I will walk around until I cannot walk anymore."

I said, "Mom, how can you expect me to be okay with that? I need you!"

Tears streamed down my face. I heard no reply. The silence was deafening.

Two days later I was on an airplane, heading back home. Mom had tended to my needs and nurtured me as a child. It was my turn to care for her. It seemed very strange to suddenly reverse our roles.

Giving her emotional support was critical. She wasn't one to cry but it was obvious to me that she was frightened. I listened and held her hand. We talked about her fears, which seemed to provide her with some relief.

I needed to be strong for her. The day before surgery, I walked into her hospital room and saw her lying in bed, looking petrified. I took a deep breath, garnered my strength, and walked toward her.

I took her hand and said, "Mom, I want to tell you that Grandma, Ron, and I will be okay."

Her tense expression relaxed. I could see that reassurance meant a great deal to her. But it was the hardest thing I've done because I knew that if I lost my mom I would not be okay."

I found myself being very protective of my mother. I assumed the role of nurse as I helped her with the breathing apparatus, getting out of bed, and holding her hand as she slowly walked the hospital halls. When she was able to go home, I slept in her room, getting up in the middle of the night to give her medicine or just prop her into a more comfortable position.

Mom wanted me to live my life to the fullest and said it was time for me to return home. It was difficult to be more than a thousand miles away from her but we talked often.

I joined a support group and quickly realized that I was not the only person to experience the type of emotional pain I was feeling. I discovered it was therapeutic to talk with others who identified with my circumstances. I met some wonderful people in that group. When I needed to talk with someone who could empathize with me, I simply picked up the phone and dialed one of the group members. They were always willing to listen and share words of advice, if that is what I needed.

In addition to friendship, I gained knowledge from the support group. One of the things I learned proved to be especially valuable.

The nurse facilitator told us that some people living with cancer undergo behavioral changes. Mom did. She had never put pressure on me in the past but it seemed she suddenly turned up the heat. There was a sense of urgency in her requests. Every time we spoke, she told me that she wanted me involved in a relationship. I was grateful that I had known about the potential for behavioral change before it occurred. Being aware did not make it easy but it did prevent my being caught completely off guard.

We shared an exceptionally close mother-daughter relationship so it was difficult not to be together in good times. It became almost unbearable while she was sick. However, talking frequently alleviated some of the heartache I felt. I was honored that she chose me to be her emotional sounding board.

In addition to our long phone conversations, we sent e-mail messages and pictures. We surprised one another with flowers, balloons, books, and cards. We shared jokes and exchanged comedy videos. Ours was a two way street.

My dad and brother were also Mom's caregivers. I needed to be aware of their feelings but it wasn't easy. Dad seemed to avoid talking with me. I felt abandoned.

Then we had an argument that brought everything to the surface.

"Susan," he said, "I can't describe to you what I felt when I learned your mother had cancer again."

As his story unfolded, I began to understand his fears and the stress he was trying to manage. I recalled Mom telling me that Dad was absolutely amazing in the way he cared for her after her double mastectomy. One of Mom's friends had marveled at how sensitive Dad was to Mom's needs. He lived a nightmare but did so with great love and tenderness. Going through this crisis again was distressing for him. He had not abandoned me. He just could not bear to talk about what was happening.

Ron did anything he could for our family. I knew he and I resolved problems things in a manner as similar as night and day. But I learned to understand him and respect his viewpoint.

My mother's battle with cancer changed my attitude towards life. I strongly believe in enjoying every moment.

"Life is short, so live it now!" is no longer just a cliché. It is an absolute truth. I work hard and I play hard.

I Needed To Take Action

Wedding plans were made for me and the man I loved. I was excited but worried. Mom had just finished chemotherapy and radiation treatments for stage four invasive breast cancer. I was not sure she would have the strength to be at the ceremony. Bill and I suggested we postpone the wedding.

"Absolutely not!" she said. "I'll be there to see you walk down the aisle."

On our wedding day, Mom mustered all her strength to be with us. She sat in the front pew, smiling and wiping tears of joy as we took our vows. I was deeply grateful that she could share our blessed event.

Two years later, our family breathed a sigh of relief when Mom passed her two year anniversary of being cancer free. Dr. Adams had told us that if her cancer were to recur, it would likely be within two years. However, four years after her initial diagnosis, cancer metastasized in Mom's chest cavity and lymph nodes. What a blow! Our family was stunned! But Mom, without one complaint, courageously began her treatment.

By that time, my husband and I had established our home in a town located forty-five minutes away from Mom and Dad. It was infinitely more difficult for me this time because I could not be by her side every day, as I had been during her first battle with cancer. Our daily telephone conversations gave me some peace of mind, but not enough to free me from my fear of losing her. Bill and I went to visit my parents every week-end and helped in any way we could.

The roller coaster ride began. Her health condition was erratic. My emotions mirrored the ups and downs she was feeling. I felt cheerful when she felt better, only to plummet when she was suffering. Anger raised its ugly head.

"Why, why does she need to suffer like this?" I asked myself over and over again.

I was obsessed with wanting her to question the medical team about points I thought were important. But my parents did not ask a lot of questions. That was comfortable for them. But not for me. I had that helpless feeling caregivers talk about. I knew I needed to do something big.

I saw an ad in the newspaper about an Avon 3-Day Breast Cancer event. The purpose was to raise money for breast cancer education, awareness, and patient assistance. I needed to raise $1,800 in contributions before I could participate. I reached the financial goal and I trained by walking many miles several times a week. I needed to be in top-notch physical condition to be able to walk sixty miles in three days. It was time and energy consuming but I was committed to do my part to eradicate breast cancer.

Walk time led to think time. I realized that Mom's way of dealing with this plight and my way of handling it were diametrically opposed. If I wanted answers, I needed to stop asking Mom the questions.

I picked up the phone and called her oncologist. I called 1-800-4cancer, an excellent resource with a wealth of information. I surfed the internet and found numerous health-related websites. Some of the queries I made, I did not think Mom wanted to consider, but I had a burning desire to learn all I could about her disease and treatment options.

I continued to talk with Dr. Adams. I asked about Mom's life expectancy, the medications she was receiving and if she was considered for clinical trials. He discussed various drugs that were being tested but had not determined a clinical trial of such treatment that was specific to Mom's condition.

While I marched forward with purpose and determination, Mom seemed to be living the adage, "If you don't want to know the answer, don't ask the question!"

When she was ready for an answer to the primary question, she asked her doctor, "How much time do I have?"

He answered, "Two months to two years, dependent upon the success of your chemotherapy."

That was tough to deal with. Naturally, she hoped for two years.

I wanted to know her thoughts and feelings so I asked, "Mom, if you continue chemotherapy for the next two years, you may become too weak to get out of bed. At what point do you decide your quality of life is more important than the quantity?"

She stopped me cold.

"Well, at least I will still be here," she said. "I'll be able to see you, your brother and dad, and my grandchildren."

When I became pregnant, I was overjoyed. But I also felt panic.

I asked myself, "What if she's not here when I have this baby?"

Once again, fear weighed heavily on my heart. I was afraid that she would not be on this earth when my little one entered our world. My high spirits drooped.

A friend suggested I read the book, *Tuesdays with Morrie,* by Mitch Albom. Through that story, I gained a different perspective of what was happening. I realized that instead of feeling sorry for myself because Mom and I had only a short time together on this planet, I needed to be thankful for the days we still had.

I thought, "Don't waste time. There is no reason to leave anything unsaid."

I wrote letters to my mother. I thanked her for all of the awesome things she did for me while I was growing up. I gathered my thoughts about her kind deeds, and put pen to paper.

As I wrote, memories flooded all of my senses. I thought I smelled the aroma of her apple pie baking in the oven. I could feel her gentle touch and see her sparkling eyes. I realized how much my mother had done for me and how she dedicated her life to our family.

"Mom, I thank you for…" My heart opened and spilled love, appreciation and gratitude onto those sheets of paper. I thanked her for the homemade jam that she made every year, for the miniature furniture she artistically created for my doll house, for our camping trips and singing around the bonfire. I told her how happy her little girl felt when she gently brushed my hair.

Expressing my thoughts and feelings meant a lot to both of us. One by one, she placed the letters on the piano. She delighted in sharing her accumulation of, as she put it, "my daughter's notes" with her visitors.

One Saturday afternoon, I was stunned when she asked, "What do you think about my stopping chemo treatments?"

That was a total turn around from her wanting the quantity of life so she could just "be here."

I thought, "You can't do that. I need you. I am pregnant. I want you here. You can't just give up like that."

But I looked into her eyes and said quietly, "Mom, it's your decision to make and I'll support whatever that may be."

She said, "That's what I needed to know."

I wondered if I had just given her permission to die. That thought was frightening. But, as things turned out, she did not need to make that call. Her body had done it for her. Her white blood cell count was too low to permit continued chemotherapy. Dr. Adams recommended resuming the treatments on a biweekly basis.

A few days later, we held a family beach party. We expected Mom and Dad to join us but when they didn't, we envisioned that as a red flag. We knew Mom would have been there, if humanly possible.

I called Dad. Mom did not want to talk. Dad confirmed she was having a rough time. Monday morning I dialed my parent's number every hour from work. No answer. I knew something was wrong.

Grandma called. She said, "They are at the hospital. Your dad had to call 911 this morning because your mom was delirious."

I rushed to the hospital.

As I entered her room, I heard Mom say, "Oh, Jennifer!"

I was thankful she recognized me.

She was anxious and tried to get out of bed to walk away but she was stymied by all the tubes and wires that connected her to medical monitors and support systems. She was visibly upset. Her behavior was like nothing I'd ever seen. She was confused, uttering words that did not make sense. I tried to comfort her.

I held her hand and said, "Mom, you must calm down—it is going to be okay."

She looked into my eyes and replied, "No. It is not!"

That is the only coherent thing she said that day. At 4:30 the next afternoon she passed away.

Mom was a Christian lady. She had a lot of faith in God and lived her life as a great example of giving and love. I believe she is at peace, with no pain or hoping for a better tomorrow. She can look down and see her grandkids anytime she chooses. I continue to feel her presence in my family. Losing her was tragic for me, but I do have a lot of support from my husband and family.

While going through all of this, my friends and co-workers were understanding and supportive. My supervisor told me to take as much time as I needed. My co-workers took on additional tasks to cover my responsibilities. I received uplifting voice mails from them at home. On the day Mom was buried, they closed the office and all attended her funeral.

I have grown a lot through this unwanted happening; I learned to let go and put my trust in God.

An Amazing Woman—That Mother of Mine

I grew up with a mother who was very strong willed and could definitely be categorized as one of those people affectionately referred to as "a character." She had a tremendous sense of humor and a fountain of inner strength. Many admired her.

Mother was forty-four years old when she was diagnosed with breast cancer. She was never one to talk about her physical condition. She held that information close, sharing with my dad but no one else.

During one of our conversations, she laughed and said to me, "Why would I talk about my health? That's boring; my friends would stop coming to visit."

I was in college when she had a radical mastectomy and I didn't even know she had cancer until semester break. After finishing final exams, I flew home. My father and brother met me at the arrival gate.

Puzzled, I looked around and asked my father, "Where's Mother?"

He said, "Now Pamela, don't cry. Your mother is in the hospital. She had an operation for cancer."

That's all he said. He put his arms around me while I cried. We drove to the hospital to see my mother.

She seemed to be recovering from cancer but within the first year following her mastectomy, symptoms of multiple sclerosis (MS) appeared. At the early age of forty-four, she walked with a cane, a walker, and then was confined to a wheel chair. At that point, she was paralyzed from the waist down.

But her characteristic strength came to the forefront. She sat up big and tall in that wheelchair. She told me that Dad was in tears when he brought the wheelchair home; she was laughing. My mother actually had this bizarre sense of humor that when things were wrong and turned around backwards, she laughed.

She said to my father, "You have such a long face. You must think you're the one who is going to be in this wheelchair".

He never got over what was happening and she never stopped laughing.

That is an example of why so many people have said, "Pamela, your mother was an incredible woman."

She spent the remaining thirty-two years of her life in a wheel chair, maintaining her dignity until she passed on.

Ironically, it was my dad who died quite prematurely. He had a massive heart attack, leaving my mother a widow in our family home. Even though she was limited in her ability to move, her independence did not waiver.

After graduating from college, I married and had a family. I taught school and eventually became a principal. That position demanded a great deal of my time and my mother absolutely hated it. She wanted me to be with her often. I was torn but I had obligations I needed to honor, so I would run in to see Mother, stay an hour and leave to go to a school function.

She frequently said, "Honey, I think it's terrible that, because I don't see you much, I have to write notes about things we need to discuss."

That was pressure!

She lived on her own until the day she fell out of her wheel chair and broke her back. At that point, she acquiesced to having some help in the morning and the evening but insisted she needed privacy and did not want anyone in her home twenty-four hours a day. She had lived independently for many years and it was hard for her to accept that she needed help getting in and out of bed.

We reached a major turning point the day I received a call at school from Mother's visiting nurse.

She said, "Pamela, your mother won't cooperate. She's bleeding and needs to go to the hospital."

I said, "Please put her on the phone."

"Mother, what is this?" I asked.

She answered "Pamela, I'm never going to the hospital again and you are just going to have to live with that."

Worried about her bleeding to death, I left school and headed to Mother's house. I rushed into her room.

She said, "Quite frankly, it doesn't hurt, so I'm okay."

Was that strength characteristic showing again or was she being just plain obstinate? I did not know the answer to that question but did realize she was prepared to die. She told me her life had become very complicated and she was ready to move on. At the time, I didn't know she had a recurrence of breast cancer but I think she found a lump and chose to ignore it. She knew if an MS patient received chemotherapy or radiation, the treatments could increase the disability.

She conceded to being hospitalized. Tests confirmed the recurrence of breast cancer. I sat by Mother as she lay in a hospital bed, seriously ill, but with total composure. Yes, she was an amazing woman, that mother of mine.

I noted the expression of concern on her oncologist's face as he entered her room. I sensed he had uncovered major problems. His tone of voice was filled with great compassion. I felt as though he was the one who needed to be consoled.

He said to my mother, "You have breast cancer and bone cancer. Your condition is terminal. I don't know how long you have to live."

My heart sank. I sat there and watched my mother face the doctor. She looked at him and spoke calmly.

She said, "Doctor, I want to thank you for how you've chosen to tell me this. I compliment you on the way you relayed the prognosis to me."

I started to cry.

My mother looked at me and laughed as she said to her oncologist, "Pamela is the crier in our family and she does the crying for both of us."

I cried again while I drove home from the hospital that evening. My husband greeted me at the door, gave me a loving hug and told me my mother had just called. He was aware of all that was happening.

She said to him, "Take care of my daughter."

I cried some more. I realized what we were up against. Throughout all of this, Mother had just one request.

She said, "All I want is to go home. I want to die at home."

I knew I wanted to take a leave of absence from my job. As a school principal, one could not take two months off work; you were required to take a full year. I met with my boss and explained my need to be with my mother.

"Of course you do," she said. "But understand, I can not guarantee your return to the same school or even that a principal position will be available when you are ready to return."

I understood fully.

My husband provided wonderful support for me. Prior to my taking a leave of absence, he had planned to retire. He rearranged his course of action and continued working, enabling me to care for Mother.

As an airline pilot, my brother was able to fly into town on a regular basis to see Mother and me. I deeply appreciated his support and also relied heavily on his wife, who came out for periods of time to stay with Mother.

Mother's need for care increased. My husband and I decided to move into her house so I could help her twenty-four hours a day, seven days a week. Her part-time helping angels continued their daily visits after we moved into Mother's home. They provided relief for me for an hour or two so I could run errands or handle miscellaneous things that needed to be done. We bonded; they were like family.

Mother was confined to bed. Even though she suffered physical pain, she continued to be aware of her appearance, always applying make-up and wearing beautiful bed jackets. She thought it important to look nice, so I had a beautician come to her home once a week to shampoo and style her hair. That always raised her spirits because she felt she looked classy, even while just sitting in bed. She was ready for visitors at any moment. Her friends stopped by frequently.

Being able to spend time with Mother, without rushing, was a blessing for me. She no longer had to make notes about topics she wanted us to discuss. And even though she was sick, we still did fun things together, laughing about all sorts of silly things. One of her favorite times was when I had a woman from Mary Kay cosmetics come to give us both face makeovers. We laughed like young girls experimenting with make-up for the first time.

Mother taught me a great deal during those last months. When I began tending to her physical needs I was afraid I might hurt her by moving her leg the wrong way or give her medication off schedule. But I let her lead the way. I learned how to lift her legs, shift the pillow under her head, move her into comfortable positions and how to handle other care routines.

She taught me to look at problems through positive lenses, to maintain a sense of humor and to achieve patience. We struggled together on the patience lesson but humor helped us over many hurdles. I appreciated her wisdom and am grateful she shared it with me.

Her humor kept all of us laughing, even on trying days. For instance, when the days seemed to be passing very slowly for her, she said, "Pamela, I can't understand what is taking so long. I guess God must be custom making my wings."

During her last days, Mother became more demanding than usual. Hospice volunteers came to her home to help both of us. They provided emotional support for me as well as caring for Mother's physical needs. My mother was so accustomed to being handicapped she knew exactly what she wanted and didn't hesitate to make specific demands.

She often made commands, such as, "Put my leg here, move it to the left. I must wear the blue bed jacket today. Hand me that book."

The Hospice volunteer said, "Pamela, Just remember, you're doing a wonderful, wonderful job for your mother. You need to be able to say no to her when she becomes overbearing. And you need to take care of yourself so you can do the same for your mother."

That was excellent advice, coming at a time when I was totally stressed out. I seriously considered what I could do to release some stress.

I did have one tool that was the center of my survival system. Journaling. Writing about my thoughts and feelings each day gave me great relief. The process itself was good for my soul. It required me to reflect on my life, where my mother was in her life process, and how our puzzle pieces fit together.

I was fortunate to have other support readily available. My school principal friends were great. They established a hot line with a phone tree. When I needed support or something to be done, I called the hot line number. Someone always responded promptly.

Towards the very end, there were a couple of very intense and difficult days. Mother became unrelenting with her demands for attention. I told my husband that I needed to go on a date and to go home for just one night. But I wondered how that could possibly be arranged. Then Doris, Mother's cleaning lady, offered a solution.

"Pamela, I would love to stay here for you all night long. I'll get up and give your mother her medicine. In fact, I won't even go to bed. I'll sleep in this chair, right here by your mom. You two enjoy yourselves and spend the night in your own home."

Our night out was a real boost. Our wonderful evening energized me; I could continue helping Mother through very trying times.

Another self-care action I took was to join Weight Watchers. I attended a weekly one-hour meeting at a place just ten minutes from Mother's house. Fortunately, it was held at a time when my husband or one of Mother's friends could take care of her. I enjoyed jumping on the scale to see what progress I had made. Trying their recipes at home was fun. Mother loved sampling the food and talking about cooking.

It was especially fun to share my *Weight Watcher* stars with Mother. It reminded me of being in elementary school when I brought home papers with gold stars affixed to good work. Written on the Weight Watcher stars were the words, "You lost five pounds. Congratulations!" My mother cheered me on.

Walking in Mother's yard was also relaxing and enhanced my spiritual connection with God. I felt at peace. Mother loved flowers, trees, shrubs, and the birds that populated her yard. She smiled when she could hear their chirping songs as she rested in bed.

In her death, my mother gave me gifts; I think she intended that. One was a gift of time. I learned to pause, look around, and see things she used to tell me about; the lone sunflower standing tall on the hillside, the bright constellations in the sky, and the beauty in the sound of a bird's song. I had not noticed those things before because I was so absorbed in taking up the challenges of being a school principal.

At the time, I looked at caring for Mother as an arduous challenge met with love. Now I realize it was a blessing and a great privilege to care for that lady, that mother of mine. We had a very special connection. We still do.

I am still the family crier. Now there are times when I cry, that I talk to Mother.

I say, "Okay, don't laugh at me because I'm crying. I need to talk to you."

I also go to her grave. It is important for me to do that, and to give her flowers. I tell her that she has given me strength, strength, strength.

I have gained a completely new perspective on life because of my care-giving experience. Although difficult, it was an epic in my life that I treasure. The blessings received outweigh any of the pain endured.

Words of Wisdom
Adult Children Reverse Caregiving Roles with Parents

"The news that Dad was seriously ill was difficult to accept. He had supported me as I grew through varying stages of my life. Now he was at a different level. We switched roles. It was my honor to care for him."

—Leonard

There are limitless challenges involved in caring for your parents. The first is to accept that you are now the one to care for them rather than the other way around. The following advice came from those who have been in that situation.

- Follow your parents' lead; let them teach you how to care for them.

- Practice patience.

- You may feel a generation gap. Understand their views are probably different from yours.

- Ask for help. If friends or relatives are not available, check with Hospice, the American Cancer Society, and local support groups.

- Have fun with your parent. They may be sick physically but they still have a need to laugh.

- Take time to enjoy one another. If ambulatory, take him or her to dinner or a movie. If not, you can rent lighthearted movies, listen to comedians on tape, look through family pictures, or assemble a puzzle.

- Ask the doctors about what physical and behavioral changes you might expect to see.

- Self-care actions:
  Ask your friends for help. Take time to do something you enjoy; perhaps a night out with friends, go for a walk, listen to music, write in your gratitude journal. Make sure you get plenty of rest, exercise, and eat nutrition meals. Join a support group.

SISTERS, BROTHERS, BEST FRIENDS

My Brother Traveled for a Cure

Nick, my brother, had back-to-back biopsies. The first indicated the tumor was nonmalignant. The second, one day later, revealed malignancy in his throat. I told him I would do anything and everything I could to lend him support.

Nick was inquisitive and aggressive in searching for medical treatments and physicians he could trust. He changed doctors several times for various reasons but his major complaint was about the oncologist who told him he had three months to live and should get things in order. That was not acceptable for Nick, nor for me. We both believed there were alternatives.

I became deeply involved in Nick's ordeal. I went to every single medical appointment with him, with one exception, his radiation treatments. They lasted only ten minutes and he said he did not need me there. He felt well enough to drive and it was good for him to do that on his own. I agreed.

I assumed responsibilities, such as handling insurance problems, working with Medicare (I marveled at how smoothly that process worked and how compassionate the staff was), scheduled Nick's medical appointments, and tracked down medical records. Obtaining medical results and MRI films presented a challenge until I was able to give the providers Nick's written permission for me to access his records.

The quest for knowledge consumed me. I searched for answers to innumerable questions. I accumulated a box full of pamphlets, books and e-mails that related to Nick's disease. I talked with physicians and a number of oncology health care professionals, including people at the M.D. Anderson cancer treatment facility in Texas. Another great resource was that of friends and neighbors who had been through this cancer ordeal. They provided referrals for doctors and told us about alternative treatments.

Friend's leads directed us towards Nick's trip to Mexico where he received medication not available in the United States. His condition improved but after he returned home, he became quite sick because he could not receive the same medications as he had in Mexico.

It was time to take drastic action. Nick had two very good friends who were cured of their cancers by a Chinese doctor. There were no promises the cancers would not recur but, at the time they talked with Nick, their tumors were completely gone.

We made plans for Nick to seek treatment with their doctor. With arrangements made, Nick told his oncologist that he was flying to China to be cured.

Dr. Manuel said, "Well, if those doctors cure your cancer, it will be a miracle and I think I'll become a priest."

As we left Dr. Manuel's office, I said, "Nick, we have a goal now."

He asked, "What do you mean?"

I said, "We've got to make Dr. Manuel a priest."

He laughed and said, "It's always good to have goals."

I helped Nick gather the required medical details needed for treatment in China. On departure day, I took him to the airport. I took care of his luggage while he handled everything else, even though he had a tracheostomy in his neck to ease his breathing.

The plane departed. I stood by the window until it was out of sight. My brother would be gone for three weeks and I prayed he would return in a healthier state.

While he was gone, I took time for my wife and for myself. I realized I was tired and needed to rest. During the months I supported Nick, I was extremely busy. The only time I took a scheduled break was once a week when I played a card game called pan. I was supposed to be a substitute in the weekly group of card-playing men but they told me to forget that "sub thing"—I was a regular. So I did try to schedule Nick's medical appointments around my Tuesday morning card game.

The physical demands on my body were the most difficult part of being Nick's caregiver. I was tired. Morale-wise, he and I both moved forward with a positive approach to each day. From day one, we were certain that we would find a way to lick the disease. We did.

Radiant Sisters

I met Joan and Marjorie at the cancer center where I volunteered on Wednesday mornings. In the midst of a dreary room filled with patients sitting in reclining chairs, connected to chemotherapy drips through intravenous tubes and needles, these two delightful, classy women stood out like the radiant sun high in the southwestern sky. The two sisters were dressed as though they were going to dinner and the theater. I was amazed at their appearance because the attire of the other patients was, understandably, extremely casual and comfortable.

During our conversation, I asked, "What drives you to dress so nicely when you come to the cancer center for treatment?"

Marge said, "I believe the more you tell yourself that you don't feel like doing something, such as getting dressed or applying makeup, the more likely you are to not do anything. Two or three days of that may be alright but any time beyond that leads to an unwillingness—and then inability—to brighten your own day and that of others with your appearance. Age doesn't matter but attitude does."

"The same applies to forcing yourself to go out and do something," Joan said. "We go to movies. We eat breakfast in a restaurant a couple of times a week and have dinner out every Friday and Saturday evening. Marge's menu selections might be limited, dependent upon how her stomach has reacted to chemo, but she still wants to go out for meals a few times a week."

Marge said, "Being in a restaurant, around other people, and hearing the sounds of conversation and laughter—that lifts my spirits."

Marjorie and Joan were unique, not just in their manner of dress and adornments. They were 74 and 80 years old but their look was that of two women in their sixties. Their vibrancy shown through any of the troubles they encountered. They looked at the bright side of life as often as possible. They were living proof that lemons can be turned into lemonade.

I said, "It's so obvious to me that you have a close and beautiful relationship. Please tell me more about your sisterhood."

Joan began.

"When Marge became pregnant forty years ago, I felt nauseous on the same days she had morning sickness, even though I lived two thousand miles away and hadn't talked to her yet that day," she said.

They both laughed and Marge joined the conversation.

"After I was diagnosed with cancer, Joan told me that she had felt pain in the same part of her body as the cancer was in mine. Hearing that was more of a confirmation than a surprise. This may all sound unbelievable but, as you know, anyone who has been around us for more than a few minutes becomes aware of our exceptionally close bond."

"Let me clarify something for you," Joan said. "This all sounds rosy but life isn't always bright. There are difficult times too. When I arrived in town after Marjorie's diagnosis, I found she was still trying to do all of the grocery shopping, cooking and cleaning. I took over those responsibilities. She needed her strength to fight this battle. There were times she was depressed because she lost her husband just a few weeks after being diagnosed with cancer.

"I have low moments too because I miss being near my children and grandchildren. But when those moods emerge, we talk about what is troubling us. We also discuss our physical pains, including the empathy pains I still feel for Marge. We even shed a few tears now and then. We both feel better after a good cry."

"And we laugh!" Marjorie said. "We are gin rummy fanatics. There have been times when we were playing cards that we were so tickled about something we laughed hysterically. I'm sure the neighbors in my apartment building have wondered what in the world that woman with cancer finds so funny. I hope they know that humor is healing and nothing makes one feel better than a good belly laugh."

I looked forward to seeing these two beautiful sisters each Wednesday. A couple of weeks went by without their presence. I became concerned and asked the oncology nurse about Marjorie's status.

"Oh," she said. "Marjorie's treatments are going well and have been decreased to once a month on varying days of the week."

That was excellent news!

I didn't see them for two months. Then, one Wednesday morning, a very special moment occurred for me. Joan found me talking with patients in the chemotherapy treatment room. I was delighted to see her and, after a warm hug and big smiles, I asked about Marjorie.

Joan said, "She's in Doctor Neal's office. She asked me to see if I could find you."

"Well, let's go," I said.

There she sat on the examination table, grinning from ear to ear.

Marge said, "We wanted to be together to tell you that I have just been given a clean bill of health!"

Joy! Happiness! Celebration! The three of us felt like dancing around the table but controlled exuberance. We laughed as we imagined Dr. Neal walking into his sterile examination room and finding a trio of women kicking up their feet and singing.

That was the last time I saw Joan and Marjorie, but those two loving sisters who lived life to the fullest, regardless of any barriers they encountered along the road, are unforgettable. I thank them for being special women who have touched my life. Their radiance still shines in my heart.

She Gave Me Peace of Mind

I was a stay-at-home mom when I was diagnosed with breast cancer and needed to undergo surgery. Besides being concerned about the mastectomy and chemotherapy, I was very worried about my family. I had always been available for my two children and my husband. Regardless of the time of day or night or anything that I may have been involved with, they were my absolute top priority. I was troubled about how they would fare while I was in the hospital. To make matters more difficult, the kids were sick.

My sister, Linda, came to my aid. She flew six-hundred miles to be with me on the day of surgery. On the scheduled morning, my husband could not take me to the hospital because he was taking my son, Alex, to Urgent Care. Alex had a fever and a serious cough. Linda helped me pack a few things to take with me and we then drove to the hospital.

Linda sat with me during pre-op procedures. She listened while I expressed my fears about the mastectomy, the upcoming chemotherapy, and my concerns about my family. She gave me a wonderful gift. She told me not to worry about my family because she would stay to care for them, make sure they took their medications, cook their meals, and when they were feeling better, she would assume my spot in the neighborhood car pool to transport children to and from their various activities.

I cried with relief and gratitude. Linda held my hand, kissed my cheek, and gently massaged my arms. I began to relax. Then my minister came to see me. He prayed that my surgery would be successful and that I would fully regain my health. I was deeply moved when Linda prayed with him.

A nurse came into my room, pushing a wheel chair. She said she would wheel me to surgery but I declined the offer. I wanted to walk. Linda held my hand as we made our way down the hall. She gave my hand a special squeeze as we walked through the double doors into the surgical area. I felt her sisterly love, and held it near, as I proceeded to lay on a gurney and be wheeled into the operating room.

The surgery was successful. I went home to heal. Linda worked in the medical field so she quite willingly, and skillfully, gave me the medical attention I needed. I had complete faith in her abilities. I appreciated the way she took care of the drains, gave me medication, tended to the sutures, and generally made me comfortable.

When she left, I could not find the words to express my gratitude. A few days later, I wrote her a letter, thanking her for all she had done for my family and me. I expressed special gratitude for the relief she provided me by being there to take care of my family. That was a tremendous gift to me, a stay-at-home mom. Her presence lifted a heavy weight from my mind.

I share this story as a tribute to my sister, Linda.

It's Not Your Karma, It's Not Your Experience

"Well, I'm glad you are crying. You've been so matter-of-fact, I wondered if you cared."

I was astounded when June said that to me. She had been diagnosed with cancer and was receiving chemotherapy treatments every two weeks. I was with her as much as humanly possible and I wouldn't have it any other way. She was my dearest friend. We did every thing together. Our friends and family kidded that we were like twins. Of course, I would be there for her.

Three months after she told me she had cancer, I was hit with another earthquake in my life. I felt like the ground under my feet was trembling and the magnitude was at least 7.0 on the Richter scale. I found it hard to believe that my mother went from being in perfect health with a full-time job and her own apartment to completely disabled within ten seconds. She had a massive stroke. I was completely overwhelmed with taking care of Mom and trying to find the appropriate medical attention and place for her to live.

I couldn't spend as much time with June as I had been prior to Mom's stroke, but she understood. When I did visit her she encouraged me to tell her about my mother and her condition. But shortly after Mom's stroke, June's mother called.

She said, "Louise, I don't want you to talk to June about your mom anymore because it really upsets her and she needs all her strength to get better."

I certainly respected her request and told her I would avoid that topic of conversation.

June and I had talked every day of our lives for thirty years. We were so close and held no secrets from one another. My silence about Mom's condition prompted her to call me about two weeks after I placed a moratorium on that one subject.

She asked, "Why aren't you telling me what's going on with your mom?"

I answered, "Well, you're going to be really mad when I tell you why."

"Tell me anyway," she said.

I said, "Your mom asked me not to talk about…"

Before I could complete my sentence, June exclaimed, "What? You know, Louise, I am not dead yet. Don't cut me out of your life!"

I promised I wouldn't but it did take another happening for me to fully realize that I was still trying to hide my fears and feelings from her. As we were conversing one afternoon, all of a sudden tears streamed down my cheeks. Then I began crying. I sobbed, out of control. I couldn't stop.

June asked, "Why are you crying?"

I said, "I am really sorry I'm crying, I'm so sorry, I'm so sorry."

"Why are you apologizing?" she asked.

I said, "I am trying so hard not to cry in front of you because what you are going through is so much greater than my problems. I am trying to be matter of fact and not show how difficult this is for me because my suffering is absolutely minimal compared to yours."

That's when June said, "Well, I'm glad you're crying because you have been acting so matter-of-fact that I thought you just didn't care."

I looked at her in disbelief. We hugged; we laughed; we cried. Our relationship was back to normal and there would be no more covering up feelings or concerns. June reminded me that she was sick but still the same person as before her diagnosis. She never let me forget that.

June knew I would do anything for her; one day I found that very difficult. She asked me to inject medication into the port that had been implanted into her chest.

She asked, "Is this going to bother you?"

I said, "My God, yes!"

"I'll have my mom do it," she said.

"No!" I answered. I am absolutely going to do it and it's absolutely going to make me sick," I said.

She laughed. I flinched as I gave her the injection. I felt nauseous and left the room.

Meanwhile, Mom was totally dependent upon her medical caregivers for all her physical needs and motion. I went to see her often. Each time I entered her room I could tell she was happy to see me. She knew I loved her dearly.

When she had her stroke I asked myself, "What can I do? How can I pay for her care?"

I planned my work and business travels so I could meet the financial needs for her intense care. She wanted me to pursue my career, regardless of the situation.

She let me know she was quite satisfied with her surroundings and the people who were always available to provide assistance with everyday functions.

Meanwhile, June was getting much worse. Each time I returned from a business trip, I could visibly see her body deteriorating. Watching the two people I so dearly loved endure their suffering was excruciatingly painful, but I believed my anguish couldn't compare to what they must have been feeling.

People often said to me, "I don't know how you can stand it. It's really harder for the caregivers than the patient."

I always replied, "No, it's not! When I leave my mom I walk out the door. Mom can't walk out the door. When I leave June, I go home and climb into my bed. I can go into the bathroom by myself; I'm not crying in physical pain. It's not harder for me."

All of that being my true thoughts and feelings, I must emphasize that it seemed nothing could lessen my pain. I too needed support. It was helpful for me to be immersed in my career, which kept me connected with the rest of the world. And I had a friend whom I deeply appreciated. We met every other Friday for dinner. It was wonderful to be with someone who was healthy and discussed normal topics of conversation. She was great support.

I discovered the distress one feels when you have a loved one enduring pain. Connected through love, you suffer with them. Many times I tried to get into that head space of what June and Mom were feeling and thinking. I finally realized I could not know exactly where they were with all of this. It was their experience and I couldn't live it for them. But I could continue to be their mainstay. That seemed to be critical for each of us. When I was home, I alternated days between seeing my best friend and my mother.

Hit with Reality

I didn't believe June was going to die until the day before it happened. While driving to the Hospice facility where she was staying, I picked up my cell phone, pressed the speed dial button to her room and waited for her to answer.

I said, "Hey June, what videos do you want me to bring today?"

She said, "Well, nothing today. The doctor said there is not anything more we can do. It won't be long now."

I pulled to the side of the road and stopped my car.

"Do you want me to come over?" I asked.

She replied with a simple "Yes."

I felt like I was going to vomit.

As I neared Hospice, I told myself, over and over, "Don't cry. Don't cry. Stay in control. Stay calm."

I walked into her room and instantly dropped into her welcoming arms. I broke down and cried.

She hugged me, then patted my hand and said, "I wouldn't feel so bad about this if it wasn't for your mom being in such an onerous condition."

"How can she be thinking about that when she is going to die very soon?" I thought.

During her last hours, she was totally unselfish and quite concerned about others, especially her mother, my mom, and me.

She said, "You are my best friend. Please stay in touch with my mom."

I promised I would do so.

Before she died she seemed to be totally "out of it" but I talked to her and I sang to her.

"She doesn't really know who I am," I thought.

I left her room so others could have their private time with June. I paced the halls of the Hospice building.

About twenty minutes later her doctor found me and said, "She is asking for you."

"She asked for me?" I said.

He nodded. She did know who I was and she wanted me to be there with her as she moved from this world.

Grief

I grieved for a long time. I reached a level where I knew my grief was still with me but it was not the unbearable ache that I felt right after June's death. I told myself that I could not continue wearing this grief throughout my life. I needed to move on, go out, do things, and have fun. Doing so helped. I still felt the pain but the weight lessened.

I am thankful for the gifts of life and joy. I honor June but I've learned I could not live her life and I could not die her death.

As a friend told me, "It's not your karma; it's not your experience. Living your life without constant grieving honors the one you have lost as well as your own life. Hang onto the hopes and positives of life. We each have our own challenges and joys. Accept and embrace them."

Words of Wisdom
Sisters, Brothers, Best Friends

It is devastating to hear someone you are closed to has been diagnosed with a serious disease. I hope that the following advice will held you deal with the hurt you feel and lend you strength to help your dear one.

Miles Apart

It is quite common for brothers, sisters, and even best friends to live in different parts of the country or the world. Travel to be with your special person in time of need is not always possible. There are alternative ways to lend your support.

- Reference the *Words of Wisdom* in *Across the* Miles, Chapter One. Tips include staying in touch via telephone, e-mail, writing letters; sending small surprises, gift certificates for movie rentals, books, or humor in any form.

In the Same Town

- Be with your special one as often as possible. Hold their hands, massage their arms. Touching has powers that comfort.

- Watch movies together, listen to music, play board games, join him or her in a craft they enjoy.

- Help by scheduling medical appointments.

- Drive him or her to places they need—or want—to be.

- Volunteer to help in anyway possible.

Near or Far

- You know that person very well. Make a list of what you can do to comfort them and make their path a little less arduous.

4

Communication

Let's Talk

His Listening Gave Me Strength

About halfway through my chemotherapy, I looked at my husband and said, "I really don't like this stuff anymore."

He said, "Let's go for a ride."

We drove to Corona del Mar where we sat on a park bench, overlooking the beach and watching the surf roll in and ease its way back out. He leaned towards me, interested in hearing what I had to say. He let me rant, rave, cry, and just generally cast off my anxiety and frustration. The entire time I was unloading on him, he listened attentively. I knew he was sincerely interested in what I had to say and how I felt.

When I finally settled down, he said, "Okay, are you ready to go now?"

Yes, I was ready. He took my hand as we walked to the car. I climbed in and strapped on my seat belt. We left the beach and headed toward the cancer center for my next chemo treatment.

Please Don't Shelter Us

After I was diagnosed with a serious disease, my caregivers, with best intentions, tried to protect me from anything they thought might add to my stress level. Meanwhile, they endured their own worries, fears, and sometimes anger or resentment about being in such a taxing situation. However, they usually did not talk with me about their personal feelings because they did not want to add to my burdens.

Although that may have been noble, I was puzzled. I wondered why they did that to themselves and to me. I wanted them to know the affect their withdrawal had on me as a patient. I knew when I was being shut out. I sensed the wall going

112

up and felt like a child being sent to another room so I could not hear the adults' conversation. But I was not a kid. I was an adult who happened to be struggling with a disease.

Being sick did not transform me into some other type of living creature. I was still the same person as I was before I had a disease. My perspectives and energies fluctuated, but I still wanted to be needed.

When my caregivers were tired, frustrated, or troubled, I found myself wishing they would allow me to offer words of comfort or advice on what they might do to take care of themselves. Being shut out placed me in isolation, a very lonely and depressing place.

I ask future caregivers to share their feelings, good and bad, with the one they support. Talk, touch, laugh, and cry together. Open communication between patients and caregivers is essential. It is a critical need for both of you.

When A Caregiver Needs To Talk

My nine-year-old son had a rare form of leukemia. That was an exceptionally difficult time for me; mentally, physically, emotionally, and even spiritually. Being a dad can bring worry but this situation was beyond me. I was heartsick and physically exhausted.

I tried to keep smiling but that was, as the Scottish proverb goes, "As difficult as trying to sit still and run at the same time."

Almost every day a friend, coworker, or neighbor said, "Gee, I'm sorry about your son."

I appreciated their concern but I could not do much with "I'm sorry." I really needed someone to talk with, to express my fears and emotions, to share ideas on what I could do to ease his pain and mine.

Friends said, "If you ever need to talk, just call me. I'll be there."

But that just was not the case. They were not available when I was in dire need. I called Joe, Sam, and then Mary. Their responses were all similar.

They said, "I'm just about to take the kids to soccer practice; I need to go to the grocery store so I can't talk now; I'm preparing dinner, maybe later."

I wished they had understood that I did not call unless I felt overwhelmed. When I picked up that phone and dialed their numbers, I was reaching out for support but when I stretched for something to hold on to, all I got was air.

I want people to know that their talk of willingness to help is taken to heart by caregivers. We have expectations based on their promises and feel rejected when they do not live up to their words of honor. Our weight then becomes even heavier. This is not to say we do not understand that they have other obligations.

It is simply a request that they try to take time when we call. Just a few minutes of conversation can relieve some of worries and lift a heavy load from our hearts.

Family Connections

Our family had little time together as we cared for our young son, but we developed ways to stay in touch. We used beepers, pagers, and cellular phones. We created codes for different situations: one code on her beeper, let my wife know I made it to work safely; another meant "Urgent—call me right away." Crying wolf was not allowed, so when one of us sent the message that he or she needed to talk, we made a point to take time to dedicate our full attention to that family member.

Technology eased our means of being connected, even when apart. We were certainly grateful to have those tools available.

A Teenager's Viewpoint

My brother had leukemia when I was thirteen years old. My parents, grandmother, and I supported one another through many difficult times. I believe I was closer to my mom and dad than any of my teenage friends were with their parents. I know that connection grew out of sharing our deepest feelings during the worrisome and fearful ordeal of caring for my little brother. We were quite a team, and I am grateful for our uninhibited communication.

How's a Caregiver to Know?

As my caregiver, Robert wanted to do all he could to please me. As my husband, he had always tried to make me happy but the circumstances now created worry and stress for him. Neither of us was certain about what to expect as I proceeded through chemotherapy and radiation for breast cancer.

There were a lot of things Robert did right. He willingly sat with me during chemo treatments. He made sure I was comfortable on those days I was feeling the effects of chemo, ran errands so I could rest, and was always willing to stop whatever he was doing and listen when I wanted to talk.

There were a few things he failed to do—but how was he to know?

Robert enjoyed hunting with his friends but refused their invitation to join them for three days at a hunting lodge. He wanted to stay near me. I encouraged him to go with his buddies. After all, he would be gone just three days and I had friends nearby if I needed assistance. Besides that, he was feeling the stress of being a caregiver and the break would be good for him. He finally agreed.

Wow! Was he frustrated when he returned home and found I had been absolutely miserable the entire time he was gone. I had become fearful and I needed his reassurance. I asked him not to do that again.

But how was he to know? I was the one who encouraged him, practically insisted that he go on the hunting trip. The worse part was that, before he left, I did know that I would be miserable. I hid my concern from Robert.

We both learned an important lesson from that experience. Communicate! Sharing your feelings and thoughts are especially important during difficult times. Trying to carry everything alone, as a patient or a caregiver, just adds to the already heavy weight you bear.

There was another "but how was he supposed to know?" moment. I came home to the normally inviting aroma of ziti baking in the oven. However, my chemo treatments were affecting my reaction to certain food smells and that first whiff of ziti floating through the air was almost overwhelming. Hands held over my mouth, I bolted toward the bathroom. Five years later, I still can't eat ziti. My palate has adjusted, my appetite has returned, but one hint of ziti and I'm immediately in a state of nausea recall.

But how was Robert to know? I had always enjoyed Italian food and the neighbors had brought us this wonderful meal. He wanted to surprise me and have dinner ready when I arrived home. We had two surprises—a dinner for me, a sick wife for Robert.

From that point forward, I kept him informed as to what foods would work for me. Unexpected physical effects from certain foods did catch us off guard now and then, but we learned to take heed of lessons learned.

Robert was a marvelous caregiver. He was quite helpful and he also was great at encouraging me to move forward. I honestly don't know how I could have made it through that ordeal without him by my side.

I learned a great deal during my bout with cancer. However, the key lesson regarding our husband/wife relationship was to communicate openly and honestly. It is no longer acceptable for us to hide our feelings, fears, or day-to-day thoughts. And because of that change, I do not need to ask myself, "How was he to know?"

Stop Nagging! Who's Nagging?

While I was being treated for prostate cancer, my wife, Suzanne, was my extraordinary caregiver. She tried her best to meet all my needs and to please me along the way. Unfortunately, I'm afraid I was not always the most appreciative or accommodating patient.

She asked me daily, "How are you feeling? What can I do for you? Have you taken your medications?"

I finally said, "Stop nagging! I don't need another mother. Just leave me alone."

She turned and walked quietly out of the room. I heard her crying in the hallway. I did not express my emotions but she certainly did. On second thought, I guess I did too. My irritability, exacerbated by my physical discomfort, flared up in a nasty tone of voice.

I appreciated Suzanne's willingness to go with me to all of my medical appointments, but when she asked so many questions about alternative treatments, I became angry. I was looking for bottom line answers and thought she was wasting time with trivial inquiries.

After a chemo treatment one afternoon, I tried to sleep, but I was restless. I realized I was on edge, worried about the barrier I felt growing between Suzanne and myself. We were talking less and our conversations seemed guarded, a far cry from the totally open and frequent talks we had always enjoyed. In the past, we had disagreements that we could settle but now everything seemed to escalate into an argument or in Suzanne leaving the room. I knew my unhealthy status was beginning to wear on both of us. Something needed to be done.

I asked Suzanne to talk with me about what was happening to us. We discussed our deteriorating communication and recognized a pattern. Under the stress of our encounter with cancer, we had fallen back into our gender-related modes of operating.

A few months before I was diagnosed with cancer, we attended a *Bridging the Gender Gap* workshop at our local community center. We learned how men and women, generally speaking, have different needs and perspectives that reveal themselves in the way they communicate. We recalled how we worked together at that workshop to build a bridge across our own communication gap. We knew it was time to reinforce the suspension cables on our bridge.

We continued to talk about what we had learned in the workshop. We even created a list of male/female perspectives that applied to us.

MEN	WOMEN
> want bottom line answers	> consider alternatives
> expect logic and facts	> trust their intuition
> control signs of emotions	> express emotions
> uses analytical approach to problem solving	> uses creative approach to problem solving
> perceives repeated messages as nagging	> repeats messages of concern
> provides solutions	> resents being told what to do; simply wants to discuss problems
> withdraws when depressed	> seeks support when depressed

We realized we had slipped back into old habits and vowed to strengthen our bridge. By reawakening our awareness of the other's perspectives, needs, and communication styles we knew what to do. Foremost, was to understand from whence the other was coming.

Ronnie Kaye, a psychotherapist and two-time breast cancer survivor, stated, "One of the major breakdowns in communication occurs when one person is in 'feeling mode' and the other is in 'problem solving mode.' Feelings cannot be solved." (*Talking and Listening: A Guide for Partners*, published *on thebreastcaresite.com* website, 2003.)

Feelings cannot be solved but they can be recognized. I realized Suzanne was concerned about my health and that was why she asked so many questions. She really was not nagging. On the flip side, Suzanne said she understood that persistent questions irritated me and vowed to pause before she shot them at me. We talked about my needing bottom line answers and her wish to express feelings.

It was time to apply our knowledge about "genderlect," a term Deborah Tannen coined during her research on communication styles of men and women. We were speaking different dialects and neither was right or wrong. Our styles were complementary, but we found it necessary to reconsider how we were reacting and interpreting one another's messages, especially while we were in the midst of such a stressful situation.

Revisiting our list every few days, we laughed a lot. We talked about respecting one another's viewpoints; recalled how we could prevent potential arguments by considering if our conversation was based on my problem solving mode or her feelings; and found that, when things began to become heated, it helped to pause and reflect before speaking.

We regained our close relationship and agreed to throw a safety net out if one of us slipped on the bridge.

Junior High Students Relate

My doctor approved my return to work, even though I was still receiving chemotherapy. I missed my junior-high students and was anxious to see them. I arrived at school early. When I walked into the classroom, I was instantly moved to happy tears. "Welcome Back Mrs. Davidson" was written on the white board in large colorful letters. I caught my breath and readied myself to teach.

As students came and went during the day, they signed the white board. I made a mental note to bring my camera to school the next day. I wanted to capture my treasured message on film. At the end of the day, I taped a large sheet of paper across the board with the words, "Important—Please Do Not Erase."

What happened during the day, not just the signatures but the communication, caring and sharing, touched me deeply. Those young people expressed their concern about my health. They asked questions and I answered with no restraints.

I said, ""I am still receiving chemo treatments but my doctor told me I could return to school. I believe I'll be fine."

One of the boys garnered his courage to ask, "Mrs. Davidson, will chemotherapy cause you to lose your hair? I heard that happens."

I laughed aloud and said, "I already have. Would you like to see?"

They looked at each other quizzically, and then moved closer to me. I sensed their uncertainty about what I was about to do but their curiosity prevailed.

Sean said, "Yes, please."

I reached to the top of my head and pulled off the wig. I heard the kids gasp. Some of them giggled. I felt myself smiling and hoped I would be able to reassure them and assuage their trepidations about what happens to one who has cancer.

As I stood in front of my class, baldhead shining and wig in my hand, I asked, "How about some questions?"

They hesitated. Suddenly, many hands filled the air.

Greg asked, ""Is chemo really a poison?"

John wanted to know if it hurt when intravenous needles were inserted in my arm.

"What is radiation?" asked Grace.

As I answered their questions, I noticed two girls sitting off to the side, whispering to one another. I sensed that they were troubled by this class discussion.

Then one of the girls, Jenny, said, "My mom and Sharon's dad have cancer. They're both in treatment now. We haven't told our friends. We're both glad you're talking with us about what it's like to have the disease."

Before I could reply, another student asked, "Why didn't you tell us?"

"We didn't think anyone would understand or care," Jenny said.

The dialogue continued for about fifteen minutes.

"How is your mom doing? What about your dad? What is it like for you at home? Do you do a lot to help? Do you have a hard time studying? Can your friends still visit at your house? Are you afraid?"

One eighth-grader spoke up and said, "Can you tell me what it feels like to know your mom or your dad has cancer?"

My students were fully immersed in this amazing discussion. I was not at all concerned about using class time for this excellent interaction. I saw change occurring in students' attitudes about disease and how it affects families. I sat back in my chair and observed the wonderful compassion that flowed forth for those two girls. At the same time, the entire class was learning more about life, not just disease.

My bout with cancer was certainly not by choice but I was grateful that my students had the opportunity to broaden their levels of compassion and understanding for people with a disease, and those who support them.

Carol's Website

We were inundated with phone calls and e-mails filled with questions and offerings to help. Friends and family were concerned about Carol, our teenage daughter, who was undergoing treatment for brain cancer.

We were ever so grateful for their support. Their expressions of love and concern lifted our spirits. Unfortunately, we could not answer their calls or reply to their e-mails in a timely manner; we wanted to do something to at least stay in touch and keep them informed about the status of Carol's health.

I decided to create *Carol's Website*. The following web pages were included on the website.

- **What Happened?**

  An explanation of Carol's symptoms, diagnosis, treatment plan, and prognosis.

- **What's New?**

  A monthly update of Carol's status, including how she was feeling mentally, spiritually and physically. As she regained strength, I included stories about her returning to school.

- **Walk-A-Thon**

  Information about the community walk-a-thon for Carol, a fundraiser arranged by our fantastic neighbors. The following month I included pictures and stories about the walk, and expressed my deep gratitude.

  (Please read this amazing story and how these dear people raised $25,000 for the *Carol Fund*. The story is in the chapter about support groups.)

- **How to Help**

  Specific answers to the often asked question, "How can I help?" Suggestions included several of those on the checklists in the final chapter of this book.

- **Contact Us**

  How to contact Carol or her family by e-mail, phone, U.S. postal mail, and when Carol could receive visitors.

- **Learn More**

  Links to the Children's Hospital and American Cancer Society.

It is not difficult to create a website. For help, check the many sources on the internet. You might begin by searching under the words "create my own website."

In addition to providing our friends with information, I discovered that creating and maintaining up-to-date news on *Carol's Website* was a gift to my self because my spirit was lifted after I put words on paper about Carol and her progress.

Words of Wisdom
Communication

According to Webster's New World Dictionary, communication is "a giving or exchanging of information, signals, or messages by talk, gestures, writing etc."

Clear communication becomes critical when a loved one, or you as a caregiver, is in crisis due to disease. Caregivers shared the following advice about talking, listening, writing, and reading gestures and expressions.

- Be available for those who need to talk. Take time to listen.

- If you are not certain what someone said or intended, ask. Disease can lend to confusion in your daily life but you can avoid letting misunderstood words magnify problems. If you have any doubts, clarify what you think you heard.

- Learn how to interpret the sick person's gestures and facial expressions, their nonverbal language. A nodding head or slouched shoulders does not necessarily indicate that person is bored or in pain. He may just be tired.

- Let your loved one talk. He or she may be fearful of what lies ahead. Be patient, listen, and try to understand his or her thoughts and feelings.

- If you sense your special one is hesitant to talk, you might encourage them to open up by asking, "What do you think about...?" or "How do you feel about...?" Chances are they do want to express themselves but do not want to burden you with their concerns. Your opening the door may be all they need to put their thoughts and feelings out on the table.

- It is important to remember that the patient and the caregiver need reinforcement from one another. If necessary, talk to your loved one about your needs for open communication.

- Encourage discussion about disease with friends, co-workers, and family members. They will learn and you will receive support.

- Generally speaking, men and women communicate from different perspectives. To avoid collisions, learn how to understand the other's viewpoint. Consider the gender gap topics presented in the story, *Stop Nagging! Who's Nagging?*

- Write letters and notes for your loved one to read at their pleasure. Tell them of your love. Describe memories of times together.

- Set up a website as a means of staying in touch with friends and family. Keep them informed as to your loved one's condition, how they can help, and thank them for their support. Mention specific acts of kindness people have done for you and your family.

- Use cell phones, beepers, and pagers to maintain contact with those closest to you.

- Hold "conference" calls. Arrange for three or four of you to talk on the same call.

- If it is emotionally difficult to talk about something, briefly mention what it is, and set a time to call back when you have regained your composure.

- Ensure you have open lines of communication between all those involved in caring for someone who is ill or disabled.

5

Incurable Disease

Fear of Dying

"Nothing works right on my body except the sensual parts. A lot of good that's doing me!"

Her comment revealed my mother-in-law's sense of humor was alive and well. Her playfulness and spirited approach to life were obvious, even while she struggled with cancer that had metastasized from her breast to her bones and then throughout her entire body.

Being the character she was, she delighted in proclaiming to everyone she met, "I have cancer."

Mom liked eating at the restaurants in the Las Vegas casinos. I recall one day in particular when she stunned a few people as we made our way to the buffet.

She said rather loudly, "You do know I have bone cancer, don't you?"

Some of the facial expressions were priceless. It was obvious that people were astonished by her candor. I'll always remember the bewildered look on the face of the casino floor manager and how the waitress, who was passing by, stopped suddenly, her mouth gaped open, as she almost dropped her tray.

Others said, "But, but…" with their words fading as they couldn't find an appropriate response.

Mom enjoyed catching people off-guard, all done in fun and certainly without malice. She did love the attention her antics brought her way.

She said, "Well, I never have to stand in line. The greeters see me coming and immediately find a place to seat me and my friends."

Her lively spirit and sense of humor thrived but her fear of dying was unrelenting. That bothered me a great deal. One day I shared my concerns with a dear Christian friend.

The woman invited me to her home to see a work of art she believed would help Mom understand the concept that death is a transition to a place of tranquility. The painting was a portrait of an elderly woman at death's door. Her arms were widespread as she moved from this earth. As she passed, the woman appeared to become much younger, radiant and completely at peace. I was deeply moved by the picture and offered to buy it from my friend. She agreed and sent me on my way with the symbolic, spiritual painting in my arms. I headed straight for my mother-in-law's home.

I showed Mom the painting and said, "Mom, I know you are afraid of dying but I hope this picture will help to relieve your anxiety."

Then I described my feelings and thoughts about the woman's change of appearance depicted so beautifully in the work of art. As I gently moved my hand over the picture, Mom watched and listened intently.

I said, "Mom, this depicts my belief about passing on and going to be in the presence of the Lord. Look at the peaceful expression on the woman's face. My prayer is that you will be blessed with peace that comes from the Lord."

She smiled, nodded and told me she understood but was still afraid of dying. She said she hoped and prayed that the Lord would give her peace and help her "let go" when it was time to move on.

As the days passed, Mom said, "I'm still not ready to go. I'm still filled with fear."

In her final hours, the Hospice spiritual advisor told us to call in the family and close friends to say our last good-byes. The house filled with caring people. Mom was surrounded with love as she was given many tearful farewells.

She slipped into a coma. The visitors left. I sat with her, holding her hand and praying. She suddenly sat up, expelled a deep sigh and laid back down.

I reached over and closed her eyes. That's when I saw the slight smile and look of peace on her face. I knew that my Lord and Savior had kept His promise and gave Mom the peace that surpasses all understanding. I was comforted by that expression, the one that will always be with me until the day that I meet my Lord and Savior.

I dearly loved my mother-in-law. My husband's sister and I cared for Mom during her last four months on earth. Even though those days were the most difficult in my life, I am thankful that I was able to tend to her needs, and through my actions, express my deep love and respect for her.

If You Lose Momma....

My mother was in surgery while I was in labor. Once the anesthesia wore off following her mastectomy, the nurses told Mom that while under sedation, she talked a lot about her grandson, who turned out to be her granddaughter.

Mom had come to visit us for a month prior to Susan's birth but while she was there, she did not mention a word about her pending surgery. When Susan was a week old, a friend called me.

After asking all about my baby, she said, "How is your mom doing?"

I asked, "What do you mean how is Mom doing? Is something wrong?"

My friend felt terrible for having "let the cat out of the bag" but at that point did not have much choice other than to tell me about Mom's surgery.

I was planning to visit Mom when Susan was one-month old. Those plans immediately changed. My baby and I flew to see my mother. We stayed with her for several days, then returned to our home in St. Louis.

My intense caregiving for Mom began a couple of years later, when she returned to St. Louis to live. I was her primary caregiver for two years, with help from my sister during one of those years. Sis decided to leave New York and come to St. Louis to help me care for Mom. She had talked to our mother every day, but when she saw Mom she was devastated. She was not prepared to see Momma ravished by disease.

My daughter, Susan, and I walked up the steps to our house. I saw Sis in the back yard. She was crying. I felt sorry for her but I was so emotionally spent and exhausted that I could not help her. I felt badly about that, but I was wiped out.

Susan, just four years old, walked up and asked, "What's wrong, Auntie?"

Sis said, "I'm upset because Grandma is sick."

Susan said, "Well, let's go for a walk."

They walked around the block a couple of times.

After they returned home, Sis said to me, "When we finished our walk, Susan looked up at me and asked, 'Now don't you feel better?'"

I was grateful that my young daughter could be there for my sister. My emotional energy was drained. I was at a place different than that of my sister. As time moved on though, Sis and I were supportive of one another and very glad we were both caring for Momma.

Mom died when I was twenty-six years old and my sister was thirty.

When she passed on, I felt the full intent of the old saying, "If you lose Momma, you've lost all."

It didn't matter that Mom had been sick for so long. When she died it was as great a shock as if someone had told me she had been killed in a car accident. Somehow I managed to keep going. It was probably a good thing that I was so busy taking care of Susan and working on my Masters Degree. I don't think I went through denial or anger. It was more like self pity.

Momma was gone and I kept asking, "What am I going to do? She left me. I need her. Why did she have to die?"

When in need, human beings usually manage to cope. In retrospect, I know I relied on two ways of coping that helped reduce my emotional pain. The first had to do with flowers. I loved the branch-like red flowers often found in floral arrangements. I know it seemed strange, even morbid to some people, but I kept a lot of those flowers in my living room. When I came home at the end of each day, I immediately smelled the flowers' fragrance and thought of my mother. The scent lasted a couple of years, mainly because my husband was such a sweetheart. He knew what the smell meant to me so he continued to buy fresh flowers to keep the fragrance in the air. I think that simple act helped me through my period of grieving.

There was another strange thing that was soothing for me. I heard a soft voice coming from the gangway between my home and our neighbor's house. It was heard only in the living room. I could never distinguish the words being spoken or sung but the sound was soothing. It usually lasted about five minutes. The first time I heard it was when I was getting my baby ready for bed. Then, again and again. It was always at night. One time, I was sitting in the living room with a friend. We were talking. I suddenly stopped.

I asked, "Do you hear that?"

I had not told him anything about what had been happening.

He said, "I do hear a soft sound, like a person talking."

Then I told him the story. He was touched by Momma's presence.

The sound continued the entire time I lived in the house. But eventually I needed to move. The house was wearing me down emotionally. It was my family home and it was hard to be there without my family. Thanksgiving day, several friends were over for dinner. It seemed very strange. The house no longer laughed. It was sad. I was sad. My friends encouraged me to move on. I sold the house.

After Momma died, Sis moved back to New York. We talked often, but there were thoughts and happenings in our lives that went untold. Eventually, we found we were on the same wave length. For instance, unknown to the other, we both refused to go to church on Mother's Day. At our respective Lutheran churches the congregation wore flowers on Mother's Day, red or white, indicating whether your mother was living or deceased. We refused to go.

I did not allow Mother's Day celebrations until Susan was ten years old. She made little gifts for me at school or my stepdaughter bought gifts for her to give to me. I was appreciative but still denied Mother's Day. I finally realized that was totally unfair to my own child. I have my memories of my mother, which I treasure. It was time for Susan and me to create our Mother's Day memories. I moved on.

The second coping mechanism was visiting Momma's grave on her birthday. She was buried in a cemetery where only black people were laid to rest. My great grandfather and great-great grandmother were there. Mom was buried near the front of the church.

One time I was sitting on the ground talking to her, telling her all I had done during the past year. A little girl, about five years old, skipped down the hill towards me. I remember thinking she would probably go tell her mother that there is a crazy lady out there talking to the grass.

She said, "Whatcha doin'?"

I told her I was talking to my mother who had left me and this was where she rested. I tried to explain it to her gently because I did not know what she knew about death, although I assumed she had been told about cemeteries because her home was located right next to the burial area. She reminded me of Susan being compassionate with my crying sister.

The little girl rubbed my back and said, "It's okay. It's okay."

Her mom called her home and told her to "Leave that lady alone."

Every time I go to visit Mom's grave I look for the sweet child who made me feel better. I still haven't seen her but I feel her warmth.

I lost Momma and miss her terribly. She still lives in my heart. Sometimes I think Susan also feels her presence. That makes me happy.

Compassionate Support

I was only twenty years old when my mother died. Even though my maternal grandmother lost her life to the same disease just five years earlier, breast cancer awareness did not exist at that time. If you had a lump in your breast, the attitude was "Well, it will go away." Mom's did not go away.

Then I was diagnosed with breast cancer. I had a mastectomy in 1978; awareness and education still were minimal. Surgery, whether a radical or modified radical, seemed to be the only option for someone diagnosed with breast cancer.

I am a survivor, twenty one years cancer free. I do know both sides of the ordeal, that of the patient and that of a caregiver. In addition to losing my mother and grandmother, I lost two very dear friends to breast cancer.

I discovered that when someone is diagnosed with an incurable disease, many people run the other way. I don't think it's because they no longer care about that person but rather it's their reaction to being lost, not knowing how to handle the situation. They don't know what to say or do so they just disappear from the diseased one's life.

I spent many afternoons with Samantha. She slept, woke up, fell asleep again. I stayed. When she was awake, we gossiped and talked about all sorts of silly things. She did not seem to want to talk about dying, so I let that subject ride.

But one day she woke up and said, "Isn't this a bitch?!"

I nodded my head and replied, "Yeah."

Then she talked about how she was feeling emotionally but chose to keep most of her thoughts on death to herself.

One of the best things that happened between us during that time was my telling her I was angry, really mad.

I said, "Samantha, I am so pissed off at you!"

I knew I was going to lose my best friend. The anger I had been hiding overflowed. I just wanted her to know, and telling her was a good thing. She was pleased that I verbalized my feelings rather than continuing to carry it around within myself.

During her final months, we had some of the best talks in our lives. Conversations just flowed and we let it happen. We talked about our families, daughters, and many things we had never gotten into before because we were always busy running around doing things. Our long talks were priceless treasures for both of us.

Samantha elected to discontinue treatment in February. She knew chemotherapy no longer would help her state of health. She opted for quality of life during her final days. She died in July.

For many years, three of us had shared a close friendship. Our trio included Samantha, Julie, and me. Even though our bond was strong, Julie would not visit Samantha while she was dying. She just could not do it because she did not know what to say.

I said, "Julie! Just be with her. You don't have to say anything. Hold her hand. Tell her you love her and you're going to miss her. That's all you have to do."

She did not budge.

Samantha and I talked about it a few times and her response was always, "I understand."

I countered with, "Well, I don't."

She said, "I do. It is okay."

I eventually accepted that, but never fully agreed. I have always found women to be compassionate and supportive people. However, we each handle trauma in our own ways.

There are many ways to care for someone. Emotional support is what I was able to provide for my other friend, who was an ocean away. We communicated almost daily through e-mail or by phone. I think I was feeding something to her that she needed—my emotional strength. When she died, I felt drained and extremely tired.

I was approached by a group of breast cancer survivors who asked if I would be on call to talk with women who were facing mastectomies. Of course, I would do whatever I could to alleviate their fears and to share my knowledge.

I received a call to visit a young woman in the hospital. She was twenty-one years old and was scheduled for a mastectomy. She told me that all she could think about was her boyfriend, who told her he wasn't sure he could handle what was happening to her. She had to face that rejection at the same time she was looking at the fear of cancer. We talked.

She said, "It's easy for you to try to reassure me. You have both of your breasts."

"No, I don't. I had a mastectomy of my left breast."

That caught her attention, so I continued.

I said, "I know I'm older than you but you have your full life ahead of you. Let me help you put things in perspective."

She was afraid all men would react to her just as her boyfriend had done. I assured her that there are many wonderful and understanding men in the world. We talked throughout the evening. That night I asked the nurse's aid to provide a cot so I could spend the night with my young, frightened friend. I was with her when she went into surgery. I was with her when she came out.

Fortunately, the malignancies were found in an early stage. I introduced the young woman to a well-known plastic surgeon, known for his marvelous reconstruction abilities. She had that procedure done and went on with her life.

I consider myself fortunate to have been a caregiver. The bond between all of us, regardless of the disease or circumstance, creates a universal connection of caring.

Words of Wisdom
Ease the Passing

As I wrote these words of wisdom, my mind and heart filled with thoughts of my friend who was nearing death. She put up a valiant fight against cancer that spread throughout her body. She continued to have a positive attitude as she neared her time to leave this earth. After learning there was nothing more that could be done, medically or with alternative treatment, she accepted finality.

Her husband said, "We had a fine conversation about walking the line between expecting a miracle and acting prudently in the world in which we are living. We discussed hospice care, last wishes, and pain management."

Her family rallied around her, gave their love, and eased her passing on.

It is difficult to cope with the tragedy of losing a loved one. With the hope their words will help you, other caregivers shared the following advice which they discovered as they walked through those exceptionally difficult experiences.

- You need extra support when your loved one is diagnosed with an incurable disease. Reach out to friends for comfort, talk with someone from the clergy, meditate, or pray.

- It may be helpful to contact Hospice, an organization of compassionate, understanding, and knowledgeable people who administer pain management and help people die with dignity. They are also a great source of assistance and comfort for family members.

- Read inspirational and self-help books that deal with losing a loved one. Although there are innumerable books on the topic of dealing with death, these three are highly recommended: *Tuesdays with Morrie* by Mitch Albom, *Death and Dying* written by Elisabeth Kubler-Ross, and *Grace and Grit*, author Ken Wilber.

- A daughter caring for her mother said, "Instead of feeling sorry for yourself about the short time you have left with your loved one, make the most of it." Write letters or tell your loved one how much he or she means to you. Thank him or her for their influence on your life.

- As a caregiver of one who is dying, you need to allow yourself time to do "normal" things. You cannot face death all the time. You need to rejuvenate.

- Spend quality time with the one who is moving towards the end of their journey on earth. Be yourself and give your love.

- Talk about the good times you shared.

- Ask your loved one if she wants to discuss her thoughts on death. If so, feel free to have that conversation.

- Offer to have a spiritual or religious person visit your patient.

- Pray or meditate together. Perform religious or spiritual rituals.

- Respect and try to comply with your dear one's wishes.

- If you believe it would be beneficial, give the dying person permission to leave. Those who work with people during their final hours say it is important to let them know that you, family, and friends will be alright, and although they will be missed, it is alright to move on.

- If you are the one in position to do so, ask family and close friends to visit and say their farewells. However, understand that part of the dying process is to remove one's self from those with whom they have been close. That is a step in preparing for letting go and accepting death.

- Family members may feel rejected if the dying person does not want to see them. Ask a chaplain, Hospice worker, or medical social worker to explain that it is not a personal affront but rather a lead into the patient's acceptance of death.

- Grief may begin before death occurs. Caregivers are encouraged to talk with someone about their grief and emotions.

- Be there to support, listen to, and love your special person during their final days. Treasure your time together. Accept that you cannot change what is happening.

6

Religious and Spiritual Happenings

The Road Between Fear and Peace

I was shocked to hear that Mom was undergoing tests for both breast and esophageal cancer. My initial reaction was that the results would all be negative and she would be declared cancer free, given a clean bill of health, and life would return to normal. Over the next couple of days, my confidence waned. I was fearful.

The day Mom was to learn the results of her medical procedures, reality jumped up and hit me hard. I was driving home from work when I found myself praying. I prayed for the first time since I was a very little girl. I asked God to protect her from this trauma. Almost immediately, I felt a sense of reassurance that she would not die from cancer. I thought things would eventually turn out alright.

However, my nagging sense of foreboding did have its roots. Perhaps some rational, subconscious thinking occurred in my mind based on the fact that Mom's sister had a mastectomy just three years earlier. Also, Mom was a smoker. That made esophageal cancer a distinct possibility and that really sent my heart trembling. The tests revealed that her esophagus was clear but she did have breast cancer.

I was somewhat relieved at that point and asked Mom, "Why are you still smoking? You have a second chance. How can you continue to do this to yourself?"

She answered, "I know you are right. I am trying hard to kick the habit but please understand how difficult it is right now. I have just moved, found new medical people, scheduled numerous appointments, and dealt with all kinds of relocation issues. This has all been very trying. I am feeling edgy and it seems next to impossible for me to toss away the cigarettes right now. I want to quit for you and I want to quit for me. Please believe me when I say I will—but not today."

She appreciated my point of view but I don't think she had any idea of how angry I was with her for continuing to smoke, even though I understood her reasoning.

I knew God was not pleased. I felt He had done all of this to shake her up, to give her a swift kick into knowing that she had the power to halt the damage cigarettes had already done to her body. I believed God was trying to show her the possible outcomes of continuing to smoke. I thought she was being disrespectful to Him and to her own physical being by continuing to inhale carcinogens.

I prayed to God and, once again, I felt some reassurance although this time it was accompanied by trepidation. I was very anxious. Soon I found myself talking with God rather often.

The surgeon performed a partial mastectomy on Mom. The oncologist prescribed radiation treatments for seven weeks. As she progressed through treatment, I began to feel that she would be alright. Following the thirty-five doses of radiation, Mom was tired but healthy.

I prayed again. I thanked God for her renewed health.

"Now she <u>must</u> quit smoking," I thought.

She did! Cold turkey!

Just a few months later, she joined my brother and me on a life affirming adventure into the Canyonlands of Utah, hiking and camping. My sixty year old, cancer survivor, ex-smoker mother regenerated her love of and zest for life. We reinforced our strong love, mutual admiration, and respect for one another. Once again, life was wonderful.

Sitting high on a beautiful cliff overlooking the pinnacles and spires in the Needles area of Canyonlands, I thanked God.

My Jewish Faith was My Caregiver

I celebrated my 20th anniversary of being cancer-free with my Jewish community of friends. Following are excerpts from my talk to the congregation.

—Ginger

Shabbat Shalom!

This is my 20th anniversary of being cancer free! For a couple of years, I have thought about how I wanted to acknowledge this wonderful milestone. I knew I wanted to do it within my Jewish community, at my temple. After all, we said a misherberach for those who were ill, we said kaddish for those who had died. What do we do to affirm health? Giving the drash and having friends bless me sounded like a wonderful idea.

At first, I thought it would be appropriate to recite the words Moses prayed for Miriam when she was struck ill. It is the shortest prayer in the Torah, "El Na Rafana la, God Please Heal her." Moses recited this prayer to God when Miriam was struck sick. He believed that was appropriate because he thought God struck Miriam sick.

That seemed the answer, to say the healing prayer as I celebrated health. Yet, when I looked back twenty years, I wondered if I said that prayer when I asked God to heal me. No, I did not. If I believed in a God who could heal me, I had to believe in a God who had given me my cancer. I did not, and still cannot, accept that. My God has other things to do rather than strike people sick. Maybe that was what God did in Biblical days, but not my God, and not today.

I looked at NASO where the specific duties of the tribes are spelled out in detail. Each had their role to keep the community functioning smoothly. I recognized that twenty years ago, I recognized the different roles each doctor had in my recovery, and I remembered praying that the doctors all knew what they were doing, that they were skilled, and that God was with them. My family, friends, and community were there as well, supporting me, each in their own way, doing what they each were supposed to do.

A few weeks ago, I saw my oncologist and reminded him that it had been twenty years since we began the cancer journey together. I thanked him for each one of those years. He helped me more than with his medications because he was the first Jewish doctor who had treated me. He helped me put my treatments in a Jewish context.

When I asked if I could fast on Yom Kippur during chemotherapy, he said, "I understand that it is spiritually important for you to fast but don't go beyond what your body tells you. Eat if you need to fulfill pekuach nefesh, the saving of a life. He showed me the path for healing, both physically and spiritually.

I wondered if there were other elements within NASO that I could identify for my situation. NASO details what happens to a wife if her husband thinks She has been unfaithful to him. The woman, in front of the community, goes through an ordeal of drinking bitter waters so her guilt or innocence can be determined. My ordeal was about infidelity in a sense, the betrayal of my body by getting cancer. So, what did I do? I treated my body with chemotherapy, the bitter waters that made me sick. And my ordeal was done within the community. In time, I have learned to understand, appreciate, and trust my body again. We are now good friends, whereas before cancer, I think I took her for granted.

I participated in the *Avon Breast Cancer 3 Day Walk* from Santa Barbara to Zuma Beach, walking sixty miles in three days. It rained the entire third day. The weather was miserable, but I felt on top of the world when I finished. Not only had I learned to trust my body again, I had brought her to new heights. I could do anything. I was more than a survivor. I made a great life for myself.

I have heard it said, "Cancer is the best thing that has happened to me."

I am not sure I would say that, but I can tell you that cancer has changed me for the better in the way I try to live.

A dear friend from Miami came to help after my surgery. She hoped that someday I would again feel that petty things were important. She meant that the cancer would recede from top priority in my life. I understood that but realized I never wanted to again believe petty things are important. I wanted to always keep things in perspective; petty things are petty and there are plenty of important things to consider.

Since cancer, I look at things differently. I see what is meaningful and shed the rest, as I shed my hair from my head during chemotherapy. Cancer helped me appreciate life and the beauty that surrounds me. I stop and smell the roses. I enjoy the sunsets over the park behind my house. I thank God for the color purple.

Birthdays are wonderful things; we all have them. Too often we complain about getting older. I am not as old as I will be. I want to get a lot older! I want to continue to grow, to pray, to study, and to open myself to new ways of living.

When I studied morning blessings, I realized that they were for ME. I was thanking God for allowing me to see, to have clothes to wear, food to eat, and freedom in which to enjoy life. These were not some Reform Social Action imperatives telling me to clothe the naked and feed the hungry. I was the hungry and God was feeding me, physically and spiritually. At the same time, I lived with hot flashes.

I prayed, "Thank you God for allowing my body to function the way she should, for helping me realize that she too has her times and her seasons."

It did not alleviate the discomfort, but the blessing put me in a better frame of mind and, therefore, I did not mind them so much.

After everything my body had gone through with breast cancer, radiation, and chemotherapy, she was still doing what she was supposed to do. She and I had come full circle and were connected once again.

I look back on the time of my cancer treatments as a separation from my everyday life. It was a time of sacrifice and struggle. The Nazarites sacrificed parts of their everyday life, to live totally holy lives. I discovered that there was life after chemo, just as the Nazarites returned to a normal everyday life after their vows were completed.

Can I truly separate cancer from my life? The cancer itself has been separated from me, but can its effects be removed from my life? No. Nor do I want them to be. I want to remember how grateful I am to be here. I want to remember all of my blessings. I want to always remember to tell those special people in my life how much they mean to me, how much they helped me through the rough times, and how much better the good times are shared with them. I want to remember that I can do anything. I beat cancer. I walked sixty miles in three days. I almost feel like the song, *I am Woman, Hear Me Roar!*

In the face of any life threatening illness, we must continue to love and say to the illness, "You cannot beat me, even if you kill me physically. By affirming life, God will bless us."

God blesses us through the Birkat Kohanim, which is in this parasha. Each of the three blessings begins with God. According to Nehama Liebowitz, the first blessing refers to the physical, the second blessing to the spiritual, and the third blessing moves us to peace, both inner peace and peace throughout the world.

"Adonai bless you and keep you! Adonai deal kindly and graciously with you! Adonai bestow favor upon you and grant you peace!"

The blessings are for us individually, but we are also blessed as a people. We are individuals but part of a community. We are always linked with one another and with God.

The line following the three blessings is, "Thus they shall link My name with the people of Israel and I will bless them."

God blessed me with twenty years of health, with a new understanding of my body and the magnificence of the world around me. God blessed me with my family, friends, and my community. God has blessed me with the power to laugh, to study, to pray, and to love. I am grateful.

Please join me in the Shehechi-anyu.

Shabbat Shalom!

The Beautiful Black Cat

My husband, Jim, and I talked about my best friend, Amy, as we made our way through the wine country. Amy was snatched away by disease and would not be present at her daughter's marriage ceremony. I recalled the day she told me she had discovered a lump in her breast.

Trying to keep things light, I said, "Amy, it's probably just a loose screw. Better be careful or your boob will fall off."

After her mastectomy, I told her how badly I felt about having made such an awful joke.

She laughed and said, "You were right. There was a loose screw and with a little help from the surgeon my boob did fall off."

She tried to cheer me up, rather than the other way around. It worked. I was relieved to know she was not offended or the least bit troubled by my comment. She knew I had been joking, trying to bring some levity to the moment.

She was also Jim's very good friend. She had been critical in helping him through his treatment for lymphatic cancer. She understood what he was going through, answered many of his questions, and provided moral support. Her care giving was a blessing for him and she was grateful to be a positive influence in his healing process. We both missed her and I was hurting because she could not be at the wedding.

As we took our seats before the ceremony, I noticed a black cat in a small alcove above our heads.

I leaned toward Jim and whispered, "Did you see the black cat up there?" pointing toward the recess in the wall.

He said, "Yes, that black cat passed me when I was entering the building, after parking the car."

We sat on folding chairs throughout the service, occasionally glancing at the cat. The black cat remained perched at a vantage point and watched the ceremony unfold. As the minister was about to introduce the bride and groom as Mr. and Mrs. Davidson to the congregation, that black cat walked down the stairs and strolled along the outside of the rows of chairs. She turned back to take another glimpse of the bride and groom, then sauntered away. We did not see her again.

During the reception, I danced with the bride's cousin.

He said, "Val, did you see the black cat?"

"Yes," I said, "that was amazing!"

He said, "That cat has been here for the rehearsal and that cat was here the entire time everyone was getting ready. We were told that she has not been around here before."

I told him what I saw during the ceremony.

We looked at each other and said simultaneously, "She's here, isn't she?"

We nodded in agreement.

Later in the evening, the bride asked, "Val, did you see my mom?"

I replied, "The black cat?"

She simply nodded and said, "Uh-hu."

We both smiled.

And I, a Caucasian woman, said, "And the cat was black."

"Yes, my African American mom wanted us to be proud of our heritage," she said.

Later that night, Jim and I agreed that it had been an eerie but very touching experience. When Amy was alive, her presence was felt when she entered a room. It was the same at her daughter's wedding. We will always remember the beautiful black cat.

Later, Amy's mother and daughter said, "She still drops by now and then."

I knew what they meant. There have been times while driving my car that I felt Amy was right there with me. One morning shortly after she died, the sky filled with dark clouds. In a most unlikely spot, right in the center of a heavy cloud, the sun shone through.

I thought, "Maybe I'm losing it but I know she's there."

I have never felt that presence with anyone who has passed away but now I consider those messages and experiences to be very important. I want to hold on to all that is connected with them.

Spirit Connections

My two best friends passed on within weeks of one another. They both succumbed to cancer. For two weeks, my friend Karen, who was the first to die, came to me in my dreams. Over and over, she told me "it" would be difficult for me but everything would be okay. The dreams stopped the day my other friend, Julie, died. At the time, I did not connect Julie's death with Karen's messages because I did not receive word of Karen's passing until two days after she died.

I have always been a very spiritual person. Friends and family members who have died, talk to me, mostly in my dreams. Susan, my therapist, listened as I told her all of this. We were sitting in her office with the doors and windows closed. There were no drafts or currents of air moving in the room. Suddenly, I was startled. She, being a counselor, always had Kleenex in her office.

I asked Susan, "Did you see that tissue move from standing straight up to swaying from side to side?"

She nodded. It was as if two little elves took hold of the tissue corners and moved it back and forth.

I said, "Oh my God, I guess it's one of my loved ones from the other side."

With that, the room started spinning wildly. I've never had an experience like that. I held on to the chair.

I must have had a strange look on my face because Susan asked, "Are you okay? Do you want to lie down?"

I said, "I can't get up."

I put my head between my legs to try to gain stability but the twirling continued for about three minutes.

Then Susan said, "When the room was spinning I could sense it but I didn't feel the extreme motion that seemed to take you. It was moving very quickly, wasn't it?"

"Yes!" I said.

Following that occurrence, I was drained and felt weak. Susan drove me home.

She said, "I won't make you go to the hospital if you promise to see your doctor tomorrow."

I agreed.

Dr. Ross knew me well because he had been my general practitioner for years.

I said, "Dr. Ross when you hear the story I'm about to tell you, you are going to think I'm insane. But I want you to know that I was with a psychologist who observed and felt what happened."

I gave him the details of my encounter with a spirit—or spirits.

Dr. Ross said, "I'll run a battery of tests if it happens again but I really don't think man can do anything about whatever it is."

It hasn't happened again but I've had loads of wonderful dreams. I believe my loved ones who have moved on to the other side are still with me. I find that comforting. Friends question me about my spirit connections.

Karen's mom asked, "Why does she go to you but she doesn't come to me?"

I said, "I don't think it's that she loves me more than you. I believe the spiritual contact waves are like radio signals. They are out there. I just happen to have the type of sensitivity antennae that allows me to pick up the communication."

I've had spirit contact with a friend who was certainly much closer to his wife and children than he was to me. I'm just able to connect with him on those frequencies.

Towards the end of the visit from the spirit/s in Susan's office I pleaded, "Please don't do this again. I am frightened. I am asking you to continue contacting me but only while I'm sleeping."

That request has been honored and I continue to lovingly meet spirits in my dreams.

Words of Wisdom
Religious and Spiritual Experiences

Religion and spiritualism encompass faith and beliefs of groups of people or individuals connected with their greater power. Caregivers often reach to these sources for strength. Following are reflections and words of wisdom they have shared about how spiritualism and or religion affected them during their time as a caregiver.

• I gained much-needed strength by talking with my priest.

• In time of crisis, we find strength in our religious faiths.

• I am a spiritual person. When I realized I could not change my daughter's health condition, I finally accepted it and had an awakening. I realized there was a greater being and I turned my problems over to the supreme power. I felt relieved and gained a phenomenal amount of strength.

• Caregivers search for answers. Many kneel to pray. Some simply talk to Spirit or God or whatever name they give to their greater power. I found that letting my worries and concerns float into the universe reaped answers for me.

• Going to church took on a new meaning while I cared for my little boy with cancer. I prayed, "God, it's in your hands." I was ready to accept His help. There are questions to which we will never have the answers, but my faith pulled me through a difficult time. Prayer is a powerful thing.

• I prayed for the first time since I was a little girl. Almost immediately, I felt a sense of reassurance.

• The blessing I received from my rabbi and our congregation is still with me. It was especially moving and it still reverberates within my soul.

• I received blessings and comfort because many people prayed for me. Ask others to form a prayer circle for you.

- When troubled, close your eyes, hold your hands in an open position, and ask Spirit to be with you. When I did so, I felt relief, strength, and peace.

- Open yourself to the Spirit that flows within and around you. You receive strength and peace.

- Open your soul to the universe.

- While I was a caregiver, I read an article that stated doctors are recommending meditation to help heal the body, mind, and spirit. I became interested in the practice of meditation and discovered it gave me peace and comfort. That was a great gift, which led to much-needed strength while I was a caregiver. I urge you to try it.

7

Personal Growth and Gratitude

A Letter to My Caregivers

I extend a very special thank you to my caregivers—my husband, sister, family, friends, co-workers, and my students. I want you each to know that you had a positive influence on my becoming cancer-free. I sincerely appreciate everything you did, from sending notes of encouragement to the major commitment of sticking with me throughout my treatment and recovery period.

It has been five years since I was diagnosed with breast cancer. I'm doing great. I feel better now than before cancer. Thank you for helping me reach this juncture in my journey.

At the time of my diagnosis, I realized my life was a mess and I had better do something about it. I was negative, a worrier, lived in a depressed state, and had little self-esteem. I also realized that for my body to be completely well, I needed to rely on holistic healing rather than strictly medical or physical aspects of getting well. Our humanness is not only in our bodies but is emotional and spiritual.

During the past five years, I read everything I could get my hands on that dealt with holistic healing. I applied what was appropriate to my life. Because of this, and with your support, my life has completely changed. I like myself now. I'm fun to be with. I genuinely care about others. I don't worry, my spiritual life is on track, and my self esteem is much higher than before I had cancer. I quit smoking, am exercising more and eating healthier. Life is so good!!!! Every twenty-four hours brings new and exciting challenges. It is really fun to face a new day. I look forward, with new enthusiasm, to seeing my seventh- and eighth-grade students on Monday mornings.

This entire epoch has had an enormous impact on me. If someone told me I would never have to worry about cancer again but, consequently, I needed to live my life as I did before cancer, without hesitation I would tell them that I'd take the cancer any day. I would go through chemotherapy and thirty-five radiation treatments once again. I would lose my hair twice again. It has all been worth it to be as I am now.

It took a life threatening disease, a drastic step, to awaken me. Today, my garden of many colors is fragrant and beautiful. I tend it with love. Thank you dear caregivers, for helping me along my road to a new life.

With love,

Mary

A Tribute to My Forever Friend and Her Strength through Trials and Tribulations

Patty and I grew up together. We have been best friends since we met in sixth grade. I always admired her compassionate and giving spirit.

She has been through difficult times, as she raised six children as a single mother, cared for her children's grandmother, and gave her time and love to numerous others along the way.

Before she became a mom, Patty had already encountered care-giving challenges. When Patty was a teenager, her mother was dying of cancer and bedridden in their home. Each day after school, Patty went home to care for her mother. I recall being with her and noticing how tender and loving she was with mother.

Years later, Patty's brother became sick. He lived fifty miles from her but received treatment at a medical facility close to her home. Patty and her husband, Al, opened their hearts and their home to her brother and his significant other. They stayed with them for several weeks. Patty and Al welcomed them, made them feel at home, and invited their friends to visit at any time.

She and Al were truly a match made in heaven. They were married less than five years when the heart condition he had since childhood exacerbated. He was confined to bed. She took leave of absence from work to be with him around the clock. She cared for his physical needs, but his (and her) brightest moments were those when they sang together.

Patty loved Al dearly and was devastated when the doctors told her there was nothing more they could do. Al passed away. To this day, she still wears his wedding ring. They remain true soul mates, in the deepest sense of the word.

Through all of her trials and tribulations, Patty was strong, compassionate, and caring. This tribute is to my forever friend, with love.

A Caregiver's Poem

"Celebration"

Judi, Judi, quite contrary
Got a lump and it was scary
Had some chemo, then the knife
Then more chemo, what a life

Radiation had its day
It was finished before the month of May
The doctor waved and said "goodbye"
And we all heaved a great big sigh

Then came time for celebration
No better way than on the ship, Elation
It's been fun with laughs galore
Here's to life and health evermore!

—Marlee Rogow

Soul Mate And Challenger

Bill and I had an eye-heart connection on our first meeting. I had never experienced anything quite like that. We had a spiritual meeting of our souls.

When I learned that he had done a lot of reading about mind—body—spiritual connections, I thought, "Gosh—not only am I attracted to you but you have all of this too."

I was fascinated by his thoughts and knowledge on that subject.

As our friendship grew, he talked about being very tired but I assumed that was due to the long hours he worked in hospital pharmacology. A few months later, I was astounded when he resigned from his position doing work he loved. He said he needed to rest. It was not long until unemployment began to make him feel insecure. He had not been out of a job since he was a child. He accepted a position traveling throughout the state, providing a week or so of time off for those in a one-person pharmacy.

We went out the night before he began his travels. He seemed very withdrawn. He said he was depressed and would pull himself out of that state of mind. About a week later, I called to say I would be up to visit. He was enthusiastic about my impending visit.

I was stunned when I arrived. He was so different! I stayed a couple of days. We planned to meet for breakfast the morning I was scheduled to leave. I waited at the restaurant forty-five minutes. Then I drove to the hospital where he was working that week. There he was, wearing his white pharmaceutical coat, practicing his profession.

He said, "I was called in during the night and have been here for several hours."

I thought, "He could have at least called to tell me we could not meet for breakfast."

I was perplexed by his behavior. He mentioned that he was having headaches but I was not impressed. I was miffed.

We continued to talk on the phone while he traveled throughout the state.

A few weeks after my visit, he went into serious withdrawal and suddenly said, "I'm just not attracted to you anymore."

After the initial shock, I thought, "This is just crazy. He has been sending me mixed messages."

But I had to accept what was. I painfully moved through the next three months. Then I called him. I needed to know why he had shifted to this stance. I could handle the brush off but I needed to understand why the complete turn around. He said he could not see me and wished me well with my life. Something told me it was all a smoke screen. Then it dawned on me.

I thought, "He thinks he has AIDS!"

Bill had always feared that disease.

I began seeing a counselor and attending a co-dependency class. Three months after our last conversation, he left a message on my voice mail. Ironically, he called on one of the nights I was attending co-dependency class. I returned his call.

He said, "Would you believe I've been diagnosed with Hodgkin's disease!"

He was euphoric. He was ecstatic because it was _not_ AIDS! He had symptoms for a year but the doctors were unable to determine the source of his problems. He talked of the events of the past year. I learned that he had lost so much weight that he did not want me to see him in that condition. He thought he was going to die and did not want to burden me. I was relieved to hear from him and to know not all of my instincts were crazy. We had indeed made a connection.

We stayed in touch through four courses of his treatment. I only saw him a couple of times but I called regularly. He was always grateful to hear from me. Things were very good between us. I thought all of this was fitting with God's plan. Everything seemed to be in synch with my universe.

However, that was not to last. During his fifth treatment cycle, complications arose. He received drug injections that played havoc with his body and frame of mind. If I happened to call after he had his medications, he blasted me. Those meds agitated him and he lashed out at me. I did not take it personally. After listening to him rant and rave for a while, he settled down. We talked for hours.

He said, "I am so grateful that you let me talk. I haven't been able to sleep for days but now I will be able to climb in bed and sleep soundly."

I could not see or touch him but I felt we were still connected and I could play a role in his life. We finally did go out one evening. That was the last time I saw him.

He was quite depressed and said, "I haven't yet hit bottom. I have a ways to go but I will pull myself out."

I accepted that he was frightened and the last thing he needed was to deal with a girlfriend. I did feel rejected but was able to cast that aside. Interestingly, I discovered that I was feeling more renounced as a nurse than as a girlfriend. I felt I had failed because I reached out to help and had my hand slapped. Then I had one of those "Aha!" moments. I recalled how I had nursed my husband for so many years, entered the medical profession, and realized that my self-identity was wrapped up in nursing. It was time to move forward with personal growth.

I began writing. Bill had told me he would not mind getting mail so I wrote letters to him. It became routine to take pen in hand and compose a letter every other Sunday. Throughout the two previous weeks, I made notes of thoughts I wanted to share. When I sat down and focused on my letter, I found myself reconstructing sentences and using the thesaurus to find the perfect word. My writing skills developed extensively.

I also read a lot, concentrating on books of a spiritual nature. Among those topics was that of soul mates. Those readings confirmed my perception of the relationship Bill and I shared. He was my soul mate. I felt that from the moment we met and I knew it was true. Robin Williams defined a soul mate in the movie *Good Will Hunting* as someone who challenges us to learn and to grow. That was it! Bill had planted a seed for my spiritual, personal, and professional growth. It had taken hold and was blooming.

We did not see each other again. I fully accepted that as being alright. I considered our relationship a journey I was glad to have made. I am grateful to have shared my soul-mate connection with him and I thank him for being there as a catalyst for my growth. I continue to search for challenges and embrace the thrill of development and progress along life's road.

8

Self Care for Caregivers

Although primary caregivers carry most of the weight, those who help occasionally or from a long distance also reach for answers to their questions about how they can lend support to one suffering with disease or disability. The following suggestions may be used by anyone involved in this journey. To ease your travels, select what applies to you.

Help Me!

Her friend said, "You are trying to do it all. I am here for you. Let me know you are near the edge, about to be overwhelmed."

As a caregiver, be aware of when your friend needs help. Let him or her know you are there. Offer moral support and ask what else you can do to ease their journey.

Sharing Caring

- Learn humility. Ask for help. It is difficult for a caregiver to know what is expected of him. Tell your family and friends HOW they can help. Be specific.

- Spread the assistance. Ask an occasional caregiver to organize people who are willing to handle certain responsibilities for you.

- Set up a hotline (or ask someone to do it for you.) Have one or two people on call for you to contact in the event you need something done. You call one person, they call others. Help will be there.

I Come First

- As if reciting a mantra, every caregiver I talked with insisted that you must care for yourself first. Selfish? No. Just the opposite. In order to meet your loved one's needs you must have strength: physical, mental, and spiritual.

- Grant yourself the right to forget, for a brief time, the trauma you and your loved one are living. Let yourself be free. You will be stronger for both of you.

- If you find yourself thinking, "I can't take a break today, she or he needs my attention," take a moment to reflect on your own needs. You need respite, even if it is for a brief period of time.

Take Time for Yourself

- Rejuvenate! It does not take much time for us to revitalize if we simply remain in tune with ourselves and pause to refresh.

- Stay in touch with "normalcy" and the outside world. Go to lunch with a friend, read the paper, converse on the telephone with people, send e-mail or instant messages. Talk about what is happening in the world beyond your circumstances.

- Meditate, pray, allow time for your spirit to rise and find peace and tranquility. Your reality will be more manageable.

- Find mental stimulation. Work a crossword puzzle, set up a board puzzle that you can add a few pieces to each day, ask a friend to play backgammon, chess, or your favorite card game.

- Laugh! Call a friend who makes you laugh, rent Bill Cosby audio cassettes, watch humorous TV sitcoms and improvisational comedy performances.

- Pets give unconditional love. Play with, talk to, or simply hold your cat, dog, or whatever species your pet may be. Pets have a magnificent way of lifting one's spirit.

- Journal. Write about your life as it is today; your feelings and thoughts, both positive and negative. Creating a written picture of your feelings is a release of pent up emotions and stress.

- Remember, you have a life too. Stay in touch with your goals and desires. You may set them aside for the time being, but do not lose sight of your personal plans.

- Take time to reflect. Give yourself a pat on the back for the great work you are doing for your loved one. You deserve many kudus, gold stars!!

- It is refreshing to be in touch with nature. Repot a plant, tend to your garden, look at the stars, listen to the sound of a babbling brook or the waves on the ocean, soak in the majesty of mountain peaks, or simply take a walk and inhale the air.

Include Pleasure with your Duties

- Music soothes the soul and helps heal the spirit. Play background music while you go about your chores.

- Read a book to your loved one.

- Do small crafts together. Create greeting cards or model airplanes. Pull out your favorite pictures and place them in a photo album—or encourage creativity between the two of you by placing the pictures in a scrapbook and writing about the particular occasion. Enjoy talking about the occasions or events.

Your Personal Growth

Personal growth is one of the great gifts of life. It does not stop when you are a caregiver; in many ways, the opportunities for growth are expanded because you are living through a trying but rewarding experience.

- Surround yourself with people who have a bright outlook and make lemonade out of lemons. The positive force field of energy is everywhere. Seek it out.

- Do you know someone who leaves you feeling down or irritable? Avoid those folks! You do not have time for negativism in your life.

- Unite with others in prayer; the effect of that sphere of influence is powerful.

- Touch someone while looking into his or her eyes. You will share a special phenomenon, reaching into the depths of each other's souls.

- Hold onto a positive attitude towards life. One patient who was his own caregiver said, "I learned that each day a person creates his or her own reality. By choice, we react positively or negatively to people and circumstances."

- Smile! Relax those facial muscles.

Fitness

Maintain your health! Find time to exercise, walk, run on the treadmill, or work out with a fitness DVD or video.

Nutrition counts! Fast food is tempting when you are so busy. Eat a healthy diet, even if it means taking time to make your own salad. (Hint: Clean the fresh vegetables—absorb most of the water with towels, cut or chop enough for a few days of munching or for salads, store them in a container that keeps them fresh.) Avoid those unwanted pounds that creep up while living on snacks or quick food. When you do cook, make enough for several meals. Freeze in one-serving packages for quick fix meals.

Rest! Try to get sound sleep. If that is not possible, at least stretch out on the couch for power naps. Even if your eyes remain open, your body will still rejuvenate.

9

Support Groups: A Few Individuals to National Organizations

SUPPORT GROUPS ABOUND

Where are those angels willing to help someone in need? The answers are endless. Struggle unites family, friends, and even strangers. There are caregiver support groups and disease specific support groups. Neighbors join together to provide meals, run errands, care for children, and clean the homes of people struggling with health problems. Schoolchildren mow lawns, shovel snow, baby-sit, and hold car washes. Friends and family members ask what they can do to help. Church groups, motorcycle clubs, volunteer groups, walkers and cyclists, to name just a few, offer their support. These acts of kindness emanate from people of all types, who are from diverse backgrounds and geographic locations. They are caregivers who ease the journey for those traversing rough roads as a patient or family member.

The stories in this chapter reveal support provided by small and large groups of people who wanted to help individuals or support a cause related to illness. They are angels without wings, who went out of their way to help others encountering disease in their lives.

DISEASE RELATED SUPPORT GROUPS

Is a Disease Related Support Group Right for You?

A circle of seventeen people shored up Jim the night he and his wife, Katherine, when they told the group that tests revealed her disease had worsened. Tears glistened in the eyes of the group members.

Jim said, "Katherine and I have been attending these meetings for several months. We have both gained strength from you. Tonight we almost did not come because we were still trying to assimilate the latest news. However, we looked at each other and said, 'Let's go. Our friends will help us.'"

At the meeting that night, Jim and Katherine felt the love, compassion, and understanding energize them and others in attendance. That group of people had become an extended family for them during their trying times; they had given them strength and moral support. Once again, individuals, and the group as a whole, shored them up against the storm.

The support group was comprised of patients, their caregivers, and a compassionate nurse who facilitated the meetings. There were also survivors and their caregivers who, initially, joined the group for support. However, as their own health or that of their loved ones improved, they returned frequently to the meetings to lend support. They were not daily caregivers but cared daily about others who were experiencing circumstances similar to those they had encountered with disease. Theirs were acts of gratitude for the strength they had received from the support group.

Group Synergy

Bob was one of those caregivers who continued to care daily, even after his wife had regained her health. At one of the weekly meetings, Bob talked about his view of strength gained from support groups.

> *"When we are born, we begin this incredible journey, realizing that one day it will come to an end. During our travels through life, there are many twists and turns. Unexpected and challenging meanderings can throw us curves. I believe those twists and turns have brought us together in this place at this time, at this moment. I know the reason we are part of this group is that all of us, together, are much stronger than any of us alone.*

—Bob Ginsberg

Caregivers Thoughts on Attending Support Groups

The reasons for caregivers' initial visits to a support group are many. Many attended the first time because their loved one asked them to go with them. Others realized they needed sources of information regarding a specific disease. They wondered how to handle day to day issues that arose while caring for a sick loved one. Some came for the first time because they were aware that they, personally, needed encouragement or assistance to face disease-related challenges.

Most returned after their first visit. They continued to discover strength, backing, knowledge, answers, a place to talk and be heard, friendship, and an extended family of people who cared about one another without regard for social status, occupation, race, or religion. Bound together by health problems, they shared their experiences with love, tears, and laughter. Life was brighter and easier because they supported one another.

Why Caregivers Attended Support Group Meetings

- The first time I attended a support group, I just listened. The second time, I talked about my disease and personal situation. They provided incredible support. I began to believe I was not in this alone. I learned a great deal about cancer, and even more about friendship and compassion.

- My waning spirits rose when I was with our support group members.

- My child had cancer. I heard about an adult cancer support group and decided to sit in on a few of their meetings. Some of those folks did not understand why I would want to be part of their group if I was a mother of a child with leukemia. I told them that I needed support to remain strong for my son. The support group helped me and, to my surprise, I helped them.

- I was honored the night I returned to the support group for a reunion. A man walked up and thanked me for the poem I had read at one of the meetings. It had a positive impact on him. Others thanked me and said thank you for sharing thoughts that made a difference in their lives. Their gratitude let me know I made a difference. What a beautiful realization.

- As a caregiver, I needed to remain strong to care for my loved one. I found an abundance of support from my group.

- When my wife was diagnosed with cancer we thought we were alone in this experience. I discovered that other caregivers shared the feeling of isolation until they attended a support group.

- It is often said, "I think it's harder on caregivers than the one diagnosed with disease or disability." Caregivers don't know what to do. They feel in limbo. They, as well as their loved ones, find strength and moral support within groups who share similar problems.

- As a nurse, I cared for patients for nearly fifty years of my life. Nevertheless, caring for Sam, my husband, with a terminal disease, was more intense than anything I had ever experienced as a hospital nurse. I knew I needed support. The support group became a mainstay for me. The people gave me great support. Even though I was a nurse, at home in isolation with my husband, I needed to know I was doing things right. I received confirmation and encouragement from our outstanding support group.

- All members of our support group were indeed caregivers. They brightened my hospital stay with their visits. One of them brought me yellow roses and a box of really extra soft Kleenex for my nose.

- As I waited for my husband to complete his medical exam at the clinic, I felt overwhelmed and tears suddenly dripped from my eyes. An angel in nurse's clothing approached me and asked why I was crying. I explained that I felt alone and had no one to talk with about my husband's condition, my frustration, and the emotions I felt as his caregiver. She told me about a local support group for patients and their caregivers. My husband and I decided to attend the meeting. We have not missed one since then. We were both grateful for the compassionate support and guidance we received from people in similar circumstances.

- My disease related support group allowed me to ask questions, share information I had garnered, and to cry. They passed tissues for criers and gave warm hugs to those of us who became emotional. I knew I was not alone. I even learned to laugh about things that otherwise could have become overbearing if I tackled them alone.

- The group meant a lot to me as a caregiver because I was able to see how other people handled the challenges in that role. They gave me the knowledge and the courage to persevere. The caregivers, survivors, and patients in our group gave me emotional strength.

- There were times I just needed to cry. Tissues to wipe my tears, hugs and compassion quickly came my way. When I apologized for crying, one caregiver said, "If God did not want you to cry he would not have given you tears.

- Learning to cope was a blessing. Through the group, I became aware of my own coping mechanisms as well as some I had never considered.

- I chose a profession that was based on giving care. I became a nurse. Later in life, I needed to care for a person who was very special to me; that was exceptionally rewarding but also truly heart wrenching. I was thankful to have moral support from members of a wonderful support group.

- I do not know all the reasons why I continued to be drawn to support group meetings, but I do know that through my involvement with those people, I saw a lot of courage and learned a great deal from members of the group. The members became an extended family for me.

- I found strength in numbers because we shared similar concerns and issues. The total gift was certainly greater than the sum of its parts.

Is a Group the Right Choice for You?

Benefits of Joining a Support Group

The synergy created by a group of people who share similar circumstances and challenges can be powerful. By participating in a support group, you will find yourself receiving and giving emotional support, sharing knowledge, and creating a bond that goes beyond any social barriers. Without making any judgments, the group allows you to share your feelings and thoughts. You will be in a place where you can cry together and laugh together.

If you do not find a group that meets your needs, don't be discouraged. Simply search for another support group. There are many available and, if you continue to search, you will find one that "fits."

Is a Support Group What You Need?

Innumerable caregivers have gained a great deal from becoming part of a support group, whether it is related to a specific disease or a general approach to caregiving. If you feel uncomfortable about joining such a gathering of people who share common health-related challenges, you may want to ask a friend to go with you. Most people are grateful to have the support gained from diverse people sharing similar challenges.

Additional Sources of Support

On the other hand, you might decide a disease-related group is not for you.

One woman said, "Although I gained support in organized groups and knew their intentions were good, I found it difficult to be around people who reminded me of my ill father and my intense involvement in caring for him. When I was able to be out of his home, I needed to be in a 'normal' environment."

It is up to you to select interaction with others that meet your needs as a care-giver. Regardless of the source, remember that it is essential to accept others' moral support and assistance.

There are many sources of support. You may find solace through talking with friends, neighbors, counselors, members of the clergy; reading inspirational books, meditating or praying. Think of how you have found support in the past and reach out to those people and sources. By doing so, you will give them the gift of being needed and appreciated.

Reach for Support from Home Base

If you cannot attend a meeting, communicate online with caregiver groups or individuals. A list of related websites and other resource contact information is located in the appendix of this book.

COMMUNITY SUPPORT

The Bridge Players

For more than three decades, Suzanne and her group of friends played bridge at least once a month. They switched partners each time and learned one another's bidding styles. However, the true purpose of their gatherings was not to improve their bridge prowess; it was to be together. While they dealt cards, they talked and laughed. Conversations covered topics ranging from how work was going, family life, to penetrating philosophical questions. Their relationship was akin to sisterhood.

As time passed, the women found themselves sharing more and more stories of friends who had been touched by disease, and how they became involved as occasional caregivers. They were stunned when one of them said she wanted to tell them something she had discovered.

Suzanne said, "I found a lump in my breast and need to have surgery."

After they recovered from the shock, her friends showered her with encouragement and planned ways to help Suzanne and her family.

Two months later, they gathered at Suzanne's home to play bridge. They resumed their card game, conversation, and laughter. They asked Suzanne how she was feeling. She told them about her hot flashes.

Their bridge game continued until Suzanne said, "Bear with me but I'm having my own personal summer again. I am so hot. I need to take off my shirt."

The bridge players looked at Suzanne, exchanged glances with one another, and instantly, all eight women removed their shirts. Suzanne laughed until tears ran down her cheeks. They all laughed as they imagined someone walking in the front door and finding them in that state of dress. They played the next few hands wearing their bras but no top cover-ups. When the feeling of autumn replaced that of summer for Suzanne, they put their shirts on again.

What an unusual and funny display of support. Suzanne told them they were the greatest! They agreed.

"That's sisterhood!" they exclaimed.

Our Community Walked for Carol

My daughter was being treated for a life-threatening disease and I did all I could to be with her. At the same time, I tried to maintain stability within our family and continue working. Needless to say, there were days that were quite challenging.

One afternoon I answered a knock on our front door. I was surprised to find several of our neighbors standing there. Of course, I invited them in.

A friend initiated the conversation when she said, "Jacque, we need to do more while Carol is fighting this disease."

I said, "But you have already done so much. You have provided meals for my family, helped care for our sons, and did housework while I was at the hospital with Carol."

She replied, "Yes we have; and we'll continue doing those things. But that's not enough. We want you to be able to take care of Carol without going to work. What can we do to make that happen?"

I was speechless. I deeply appreciated all the help they had already given. I could not get over the fact that they wanted to do still more.

They said they had formed a committee to generate ideas and lay out a plan. The first thing they discovered in their brainstorming session was that whatever project they undertook would need to include children. That was not surprising because our community focused on families.

But I was astounded when one of them said, "We want to have a fundraiser, a walk-a-thon to raise money for *The Carol Fund*."

I told them I thought they were phenomenal people and their love and caring continued to sustain us; but to arrange a fundraiser? I needed to give that some thought.

Initially I was hesitant because I was not sure how I felt about my entire world knowing that I was faced with financial problems. I had always been self-reliant. I did not know how to handle their offer. After some soul-searching, I faced reality. My most important commitment was to help Carol. If I could be home rather than at work, it would be possible for me to care for her physical needs and to be able to just sit with her when she needed comforting. I would be able to overlook a little household clutter, prepare food she could eat without becoming nauseous, and be available to help her through difficult times. On top of that, I could still care for the rest of my family. What a treasured gift for my daughter, her brothers, my husband, and myself.

I agreed to the walk-a-thon.

In just three weeks, our marvelous neighbors pulled it all together. The walk-a-thon became their mission. They were organized! They prepared road signs, gathered sponsors, provided a journal for walkers to write messages to Carol, recruited a volunteer nurse to be on the trail, and arranged for safety measures throughout the route. These people were gifted, talented, and loving, men and women committed to the residents of their community.

I did not want this to become a "sensational" news story. There were many children facing the cancer challenge, not just Carol. The event organizers respected my wishes and advertised only through word of mouth and by distributing flyers at our local schools.

At three o'clock on the scheduled Sunday morning, the thunder clashed like symbols. Lightning bolted through the sky. I was wide-awake. I lay in bed and thought perhaps no more than thirty people, committee and close friends, would show up during this inclement weather. I thought how wonderful it would be if they walked for us, especially in this bad weather.

By four a.m., I was out of bed. I dressed, prepared breakfast, and laid out rain gear for my family. My husband and children dressed, ate breakfast, looked out the window and wondered what the day held. I was truly amazed when the rain stopped at six a.m. The sky cleared and "Minnesota humid" surrounded us. It was hot and muggy. Then, I wondered if anyone would want to walk in that kind of heat.

I was flabbergasted when over five-hundred people appeared at the walk-a-thon starting point by 8:30 a.m. Five hundred! It was an unbelievable display of support.

The parade of walkers made their way through the streets of our town. It was a beautiful expression of love and caring. And, they had such a good time as they walked, talked, laughed, sang, pushed baby strollers, and even skipped with their children. Carol and I were deeply touched.

A few days later, the neighborhood committee presented us with a check for $25,000! I was completely overwhelmed with emotions and gratitude.

I was able to quit my job and be home for Carol. I will be forever grateful to my neighbors and friends for their love, incredible acts of kindness, and extraordinary support.

Woodgate Neighbors Race for the Cure

Three months after my mom was diagnosed with breast cancer, she saw an ad for the *Susan G. Komen Race for the Cure.* I was only ten years old but had learned some about the disease called breast cancer so when Mom asked if I would like to walk a 5K with her, I was excited. We decided to ask a few of our neighbors to join us. The first year, five of us walked together. Afterwards, our enthusiasm and commitment was contagious. Word of the event and cause spread throughout our neighborhood.

The "race" is held in Minneapolis each Mothers' Day. In January of the second year, our neighbors began talking about the event and scheduled it on their calendars. Three months in advance, they registered as a team. They were especially interested in participating because they wanted to support Mom. Twenty of us walked together. We wore signs in honor of Mom and others we had come to know who had the same disease.

That was simply the beginning of something wonderful. By the fifth year, fifty-six men, women, and children from our neighborhood made the journey together. Rain or shine, we have walked in the Minneapolis *Race for the* Cure on every Mothers Day since the first year when a few neighbors joined Mom and I as an expression of their support for my mother and all who have suffered with breast cancer. The event became an all day happening as our neighbors decided to go to the park or gather at someone's home following the race. We are all fortunate to live in our Woodgate neighborhood and to be part of this close-knit group.

After Eight Years,
I Found My Support Group

As a police officer in the line of duty, and in self defense, I shot a man. I killed him. I was frozen in the moment. I had just taken life from a human being. It did not matter to me that it was self defense or that I knew it might happen someday. When the lieutenant appeared on the site, I was absolutely stunned by his words.

He looked at me and asked, "Where is your hat?"

"What? What do you mean where is my hat?" I thought. I just killed a man and you ask about my hat? Why not ask if I am alright?"

I hurt deeply. I did not leave the police force at that time but I did carry a heavy weight with me for several years.

I told my wife repeatedly, how sad I continued to feel about taking a man's life. Even though she was my best friend and would die for me, she just did not get it; she never quite understood the essence of my pain. I wanted to tell another cop. I wanted to tell someone who had been in the trenches or, for whatever reason, could understand my grief at its deepest level. But I did not know where to turn. There were no support groups for cops. It was the seventies and men were expected withhold expressions of their feelings and concerns. We needed to be macho.

My wife thought I could find strength and encouragement at church. After trying several Catholic churches in our city, we went to one more. It happened to be a predominantly black congregation. I'm Caucasian. I love gospel music. I'm a drummer. I was the only white guy in a band composed of black men in the military. I liked the gospel music at the church and I liked the friendly people.

We attended the church regularly for a couple of months, yet I was still feeling strange about the congregation being so nice to me. I felt like I was living a lie; as though I had done something to their families and yet, every Sunday I accepted their warmth and caring.

On Pentecost Sunday, we arrived to find the priest had the chairs all turned backwards.

He said, "Today we are going to do something different. Instead of a sermon, I'm asking you to tell how the Lord has worked in your life."

A woman in the third row stood up and told about the joy she felt when her granddaughter was born; a man rose and said he was thankful that his son had fully recovered from serious injuries that result from an accident. As the congregation members spoke, I felt myself wanting to rise and "let it all out."

But when someone else stood, I thought, "Good, I cannot speak now."

Finally, I forced myself to my feet. I was bawling like a child but somehow the words made it out through my quivering lips.

I said, "I can't stand coming to church here any longer until I tell you something that gives me great pain. I killed a black person. I am a police officer. He tried to shoot me. I shot him. I cannot handle your being so nice to me and my family."

I sat down, sobbing. My children looked at me with anxious eyes, wondering what had just happened.

As soon as the mass was over, I headed for the nearest exit. When I stepped outside, half the congregation surrounded me. They spoke of their gratitude for police officers who guarded their community. They thanked me for being a police officer and told me they were happy I was attending their church. I walked out of church that day feeling as high as a kite lifted by the winds of love.

My family and I continued attending the church with the congregation that allowed me into their hearts and provided the support I so terribly needed. Within three months, I was a drummer with the gospel choir.

After carrying such a heavy burden for eight years, I found my support group.

National Fundraisers
as
Life-Altering Events

Numerous disease-related organizations hold fundraisers to create awareness and raise money for research, education, and treatment of specific illnesses. Each one is of great value for those suffering with a disease or disability, as well as for those who care about finding a cure and supporting someone they know with a specific health problem.

The following stories are about caregivers and survivors who walked sixty miles in three days, committed to doing their part to help eradicate breast cancer. In order to participate, they were required to raise a minimum of $1,800 for the breast cancer cause and to train their bodies so they would be in tip-top physical condition to make the trek.

The journeys were physical feats for most of them, but their rewards were immeasurable. It seems that all were touched in some special way; many found the events to be life changing.

Here are their stories.

Why We Walk

A "walker coach" wrote the following letter to her group of people training for a sixty mile walk over a period of three days. The purpose of the event was to raise awareness of and monies for breast cancer research and community outreach programs.

Hello team—

As you know, I normally write with great enthusiasm and boundless energy. I'm sorry to say that today I'm not myself and I know that will be reflected in the tone of this e-mail. For that, I am sorry. I want to share a story with you.

On March 7, I spoke with one of my walkers, Monica, for the first time. She told me that she was a thirty-year old breast cancer survivor. She finished chemotherapy and radiation a few months earlier and her New Year's resolution was to be strong enough to walk in the *Avon Breast Cancer 3 Day* event in October.

April 12th, Monica sent an e-mail asking me to pray for her. She said she was very scared because she had just been told the results of an MRI that revealed three small metastases brain tumors. She was scheduled for a biopsy of two swollen lymph nodes the following day. Things got worse from that point on but please excuse me for choosing not to elaborate on the specifics of her condition.

May 9th, Monica wrote, "Although one doctor has given me a worst case scenario of only six months, my doctor has a patient who has been in treatment for over four years. I spoke to her and you would never know she has cancer! I am hoping to be just like her!"

Monica was filled with hope.

A few weeks ago, I learned through another walker that Monica was on life support. I went to visit her in the hospital just a few hours after the medical team had moved her from the intensive care unit into her hospital room. She was very happy to see me—it was the first time we had met face to face. She looked nothing like the picture she had sent me months earlier, which was taken on her wedding day just one year ago.

It was apparent that the disease was ravaging her body but her mind was strong and her spirits were high. She still talked of walking in the Avon 3 Day event for breast cancer.

Last night I received heartbreaking news. Monica passed away early Sunday morning, just a few weeks after her 31st birthday.

I am sharing this story to remind you why we are walking; to remind you of the devastating effects of this disease; to remind you that breast cancer doesn't discriminate. Monica was one of us. We are walking for Monica, for those who continue to fight, and in memory of others who have lost the battle.

There are no words that could fully describe how passionate Monica was in her desire to walk. In the last e-mail I received from her she wrote, "I don't know if I will be able to walk very far in the *Avon 3 Day* event. Is it ok if I only walk a few miles?"

I ask you to help keep her spirit alive by thinking of Monica any time you feel like giving up, when you feel you can't continue training, whenever you feel tired or sore or overwhelmed.

Monica showed enormous strength of character in the face of tremendous adversity and I will always admire her for that. As much as I am grieving right now, I feel lucky that I was fortunate enough to know Monica, even if only for a brief period. She was very special and touched many lives.

Perhaps on your three-day journey you can derive strength from Monica's beautiful spirit. I know she will be there, spiritually, with all of us. I just wish she could be there physically.

This is why we walk. Some day there will be a world in which we won't lose our beautiful mothers, daughters, sisters and wives to such an awful disease.

Take care of yourselves. I'll see you soon.

Nancy

2 Feet—3 Days—60 Miles

It was an incredible journey filled with moments ranging from sheer exhilaration to those of complete exhaustion. With my daughter by my side, we walked sixty miles in three days. We laughed, we cried, we hugged. Our legs ached and our feet were sore but we were determined. This journey with 3,150 other dedicated women and men who were committed to raising awareness of breast cancer and dollars to fight this disease, was important to us and an infinite number of others who would benefit from our efforts. Thousands of people lined the streets of California coastal towns between Santa Barbara and Malibu. Along the way, the random acts of kindness from those cheerleaders on the sidewalks and among the walkers themselves created an almost unbelievable bond between a myriad of widely diverse people.

Several months prior, I had seen an ad for the Avon breast cancer 3-day event. I immediately called Katie, my daughter.

I told her about it and said, "Let's do this together!"

Without a moment's hesitation, she enthusiastically replied, "Absolutely!"

We both wanted to make a difference in the fight against breast cancer.

With great anticipation, I began training. Walking sixty miles in three days meant I needed to get into shape. The encouragement I received from my husband, friends and family provided that extra spark I needed when frustration set in, which happened when it seemed that all I was doing with my life was walking. 116-degree heat during the summer in Las Vegas meant walking at 5:30 a.m. I guzzled gallons of water and on several days looked and felt like a "drowned rat" after three or four hours of putting one foot in front of the other. My goal was to walk at least fifteen miles and be able to do so again the next day.

All those miles and hours added up. The first time I completed three miles I had a sense of accomplishment. However, that was just the beginning. A couple of months later I walked nine and twelve miles a day and was overjoyed. But, the day I walked 16.8 miles of hills I felt exhilarated. I knew I had reached my goal. Three pair of running shoes and numerous miles under my belt, I was ready.

There was more to preparing than getting into physical shape. There was the challenge to raise a minimum of $1,800. Could I achieve that goal? I had no idea that road would become so poignant. I cried tears of joy and gratitude as I received pledges from my family and friends. I was touched by their generosity and strong support of my efforts to make this walk and for all of us to do our part to eradicate this disease. Their generosity took me beyond the required $1,800 goal.

I submitted the pledges and completed training. The time was drawing close. The day before the event, America West flight #497 arrived at McCarran Airport on time. Katie disembarked with her usual sparkle and we both bounced through the concourse. We were excited and didn't know if we could get any sleep that night. It was already 10:15 p.m. We needed to be on the road by 6:00 a.m. to drive from Las Vegas to Santa Barbara.

We arrived at the event site, Chase Palm Park, by 3:00 pm, where we joined thousands of others standing in the rain to complete the registration process.

The incredible journey began the next morning. Still dark, standing in a muddy field awaiting kick-off time, we felt damp and cold physically but spiritually we were as warm as sunshine. We listened to speakers and felt the presence of electric excitement all around us. Over 3,000 people inhabited that patch of land by the sea, anxiously awaiting the "GO!" announcement. With a deafening cheer, we began.

During the Day Zero opening ceremony, the president of the organization that arranged the entire event, asked us to look at the upcoming three days through the eyes of our childhood. Remembering when we were young, we recalled the feeling of complete trust and faith in others. We thought of times when kindness was given freely, with no expectations of anything in return. He asked us to approach the upcoming journey with that sense of kindness. The amazing thing is that it worked! Over 4,000 people, including the crew and volunteers, showed that kindness is like a baby; it grows fast.

We paraded through neighborhoods where residents had set up their own cheering sections.

"You are so beautiful. You look like a rainbow. Thank you for walking," shouted several senior citizens who stood on their balcony, smiling and waving to us.

Children gave us candy, jumped up and down, and waved their pom-poms as they did cheers they had created just for this occasion. People clapped, gave high five hands, and called out, "Thank you." They chanted, "heroes, heroes, heroes".

Near the finish line on Day 3, a woman who was seated in a chair on the sidewalk, shouted, "You go girls!"

The sign she held whispered a heart-wrenching message: "I have breast cancer again. You are my hope."

My heart swelled while tears streamed down my cheeks, blending in with the raindrops. We were all fighting this dreadful disease. The walkers were actively doing something that day but we were not alone. Everyone along that route was enveloped in the spirit of winning the fight. Those people and our friends and family were with us for as many personal reasons as there were supporters.

The crew and volunteers were incredible with their happy faces, songs, costumes, and numerous acts of kindness. There was "smiley guy" who kept appearing along the walk handing out smiley faces, holding up his smiley signs, applauding us, and just generally making Katie, me, and everyone else curve our lips upward and feel good. Butterfly man, dressed as his namesake, rode his bike back and forth, ensuring the safety of the walkers and checking to see if anyone needed anything. The bikers in their leather jackets and wearing welcoming smiles were dedicated to their jobs of making sure traffic gave right of way. The 525 crew members fed us, set up the campsites, provided medical services for sore backs, blistered feet, and aching muscles. Kindness abounded.

Everyone involved in the event kept us going even when the going got really tough on Day 3 as we walked the Santa Monica hills along the Pacific Ocean on Highway One. The rain and the wind were brutal that day. I was determined to endure the elements. Later, I was told that several of the walkers had been taken to the hospital and treated for hypothermia. Because we were given an inaccurate weather report, most of us were not dressed for the inclement weather. We were grateful when we received Mylar blankets along the route; another thoughtful act of the crewmembers. We tried to anchor these warming wraps around our shivering bodies. Some walkers wore trash bags. We looked like a community of aliens who had assumed control of the Pacific Coast Highway.

During the entire sixty mile trek, my most difficult moment came on that final day. Katie, suffering from a tendon injury, began to have difficulty walking on Saturday. After a chiropractor in camp treated her that night, her pain dissipated quite a bit. She was determined to walk across that finish line! However, the chiropractor's prognosis was accurate. Not only did the pain in her right knee and thigh recur but also her left leg joined in giving her pain. I was so afraid that if she continued walking the result would be a long term injury. She finally made the extremely difficult decision that she could not walk the remaining eleven miles.

I wanted to stay with her. I told her I could not leave her alone.

With tears on her cheeks but a laugh in her voice, she replied, "Alone? Mom, I am with 3,000 other people. I will be safe."

That being true it was still tough to leave her while she was in pain.

She insisted, "Mom—go now! Don't wait any longer or you will be swept. (Swept meant a van would come by and pick up straggling walkers who would then be transported to the closing ceremony.) You have been training for this walk for months. It is important for you to cross the finish line. Go!"

After many hugs and lots of tears, I walked on, looking back, missing having Katie by my side. We each had to accept that we were taking the right actions.

She hobbled along, her tears washed by the raindrops. Katie was hurting physically and emotionally. Mentally, she knew she had made the right decision.

Later she said, "Mom, I thought, 'After all, if Mark McGuire was out for a season due to the same type of TI band injury, it could happen to anyone.'"

None of this rationale alleviated her anguish. Later, in the medics' tent, she came to peace and accepted that she had done her best. She raised the monies to help fight breast cancer and she walked fifty miles to demonstrate her commitment to the cause and to support her mom.

As I continued walking, I noticed again how people checked on one another to see if any help could be offered. Meanwhile, Katie was experiencing kindness around her. She tried to warm herself with a blanket when a medic walked up and helped tuck the fleece around her. She was grateful.

She said, "Another medic walked right up to me and handed me a cup of hot tea. He did not even question if I needed anything.

He simply handed it to me as he said, "Here, this is for you."

I sighed my sincere thanks. Then they brought us chili; even vegetarian chili for us green wristband wearing walkers. I could not believe it. The crew thought of every detail to meet our needs. Kindness, without even a brief flash of expectation for anything in return. I loved being with people who gave and accepted kind acts. I could offer kindness without being questioned. That was wonderful."

Crossing the finish line, my body was tired but my spirit was jubilant. It was still raining as the 3,000 walkers headed towards the area where the closing ceremony was to be held. We were soaked through to the bone. Our silver Mylar sheets, trash bags, and colorful hooded rain jackets shielded our bodies somewhat from the cold. What a sight to behold. The spectator bleachers and surrounding grounds were filled with people. Walkers and spectators formed a wide aisle for those of us wearing pink shirts under their rain gear, the breast cancer survivors.

I was filled with joy and overwhelmed with emotion as I walked down that aisle formed by thousands of people.

They cheered for the breast cancer survivors, gave the thumbs-up sign, reached out to share a high-five, and shouted, "Heroes! You did it! Thank you."

I was moved by the direct eye contact and compassion I felt from each of these supportive individuals.

At the very same moment that we survivors entered the ceremonial area, the rain stopped and the sun peaked out from behind the clouds to shine upon the wondrous crowd of people who were sharing their commitment to beating breast cancer. I spotted Katie cheering and waving. We hugged and I sobbed again. My feelings of joy were spilling over.

Over 4,000 people gathered on Zuma Beach that afternoon. The ground was dimpled with numerous pockets in the sand, each filled with about two inches of rain. Compassion and love radiated throughout the colorful, soaked crowd, giving us warmth. As I looked at the Pacific Ocean, I gasped in awe. The surf was breaking within a few feet of the beach. Swimming, right there at the edge of the surf, were four dolphins!

I Walked to My Epiphany

The experience was life-changing for me. I walked sixty miles in three days to support my mother, a fifteen year breast cancer survivor. I raised $1,800 for breast cancer research and education. In return, I received a tremendous unexpected gift: an awakening.

Walkers and crewmembers filled the days with random acts of kindness. Compassion shone in the sun and, on day three, through the rain. The experience reinforced my faith in humanity and gave me a greater sense of purpose.

The magic of sharing commitment to a cause was a bond among 3,000 people, most of who were meeting one another for the first time. It was a big challenge to keep walking with sore feet and strained muscles but the journey was magical.

I vowed to walk again the following year with my mother by my side, but that plan was obliterated. Once again, Mom was diagnosed with breast cancer. A month later, I supported her again by walking another sixty miles and raising another 1,800 dollars. I participated in the same event, held in a different city.

The experience was a powerful reminder that I wanted to do something meaningful with my life. Before mom was diagnosed, I had been working in a field that seemed to me to be lacking a significant purpose. I hated going to work. I felt like I was making a difference in no one's life. Career wise, I felt empty. After mom's diagnosis, I gave up that six year career and took a decrease in pay to become a walker coach for the organization that arranged those sixty mile fundraising events. My job was to assist walkers during their preparation and training for the event. I spoke with them on the phone, met many in person, communicated through e-mail, and gave words of advice and lots of encouragement. I felt I made a difference in many lives. My mother loved what I was doing. She was quite proud of me. She knew I was committed to my work.

A real plus of the three day events was the different spin placed on the challenge of winning the battle against breast cancer. Walking those sixty miles provided an outlet and gave people a sense of empowerment. Their efforts were strong messages of support for their friends and loved ones who had lived with this dreadful disease; and many, with determination to try to eradicate breast cancer, walked in memory of a loved one.

I asked my parents if they would like to participate as crewmembers in one of the events. They were delighted and excited about the opportunity to contribute to the cause, as well as having a chance to be part of what I was doing. Mom and Dad worked at a pit stop, handing out food to walkers. They were completely involved with all that happened around them. They experienced the community that evolved among three thousand walkers and five hundred crewmembers, in a mere three days. They were moved to tears by things people said or did.

I received an e-mail from a dear friend who had volunteered to crew as manager of traffic control at one of the events.

He wrote, "This is the heartbreaking story I've received from one of my crew members. I'm getting many stories that share the same thread of sadness."

The story read, "I was scheduled to do traffic control last year on the three-day walk but on the morning of Day One, my wife was hospitalized. A few months later she died of breast cancer. I was married to her for forty-two years. I miss her so much."

Another memoir was that of a thirty-year old man who lost his young wife to breast cancer. They had been together eleven years. How did he handle this? I don't know.

It was hard not to become overwhelmed by the amount of suffering cancer brought to people, patients, and their caregivers. With all the thought and tears I've experienced concerning the pain and horror of this disease I have also amazed myself by being able to maintain some equilibrium. I worked at maintaining my personal balance.

One of my walkers lost her life to cancer before the scheduled event. Via e-mail, I told her story to the rest of my walking team. I immediately received e-mail messages from walkers who thanked me for helping them realize why they were training, feeling aches and pains, as they walked in preparation for one of the most rewarding times they would experience in their lives.

Knowing I made a difference and helped people understand that our day to day problems were minuscule in the great scheme of things, led to my self knowledge that I was doing something important.

I loved my job! It gave me the opportunity to make a difference in other's lives. Sometimes all I could do was listen, allowing others to express their feelings, fears and joys. There were times I believed I was a sounding board. Other times I felt like a valve that others could open to release steam, and their tears. My job was all about people.

Death of one of my walkers was difficult for me. I was not myself for quite a while. We had shared many conversations but I only met her in person once. That was shortly before she passed on. However, I felt very close to her. She was truly a special person. She wanted to live so badly, and she wanted to walk in the upcoming *Avon 3 Day* event for breast cancer. That is one of the examples of how my job was tough at times. However, it was also healing to be in that environment.

Becoming a walker coach was one of the best things I have done in my life. I was committed to the cause and had deep compassion for those living with cancer, as well as for their caregivers who suffer right along with them.

The walkers and crewmembers that experienced the *Avon 3 Day*, left the journey with new inner strength and a deeper connection with others who shared dedication to gaining ground against cancer. They walked away with a desire to instill in others the meaning of the Pallotta TeamWork's year 2000 slogan:

human**kind**

(be both)

Could Not Have Happened Over a Cup of Coffee

I walked for Amy, my soul friend, who lost her life to cancer. How I missed her! She was a woman who brought light into a room by her mere presence. She commanded attention because she was very warm, vivacious, gracious, and full of life. In her memory, I raised $1,800 for the breast cancer cause.

My thoughts and love were also with my husband and daughter, both living daily with the thought that their cancers could recur. I trained for months so I could walk sixty miles in three days in their honor.

Compassion abounded on the streets as we walked and talked. I was amazed at the depths of the conversations between people who had just met. We shared thoughts we would not have touched over a cup of coffee. I have never been exposed to an environment with that level of caring. I wished people throughout the world could see and feel the benefit of kindness and sincere caring.

As I walked, the muscles in the back of my legs tightened. I bent down to stretch my legs.

I heard someone ask, "Are you okay?"

I looked up and burst into tears. I saw my girlfriend whom I had not seen for a couple of years; since we had a falling out. We had a mother-daughter type of relationship but something occurred that created a chasm between us. We had not spoken since that break.

She said, "I heard you were going to be participating in this walk. I decided I was going to search for you."

"A friend told me you would be walking and I was determined to find you," I said.

We both laughed. The next two nights in camp, I made a point of being in contact with her. I knew our relationship would not be what it was in the past but at least we dropped the bitterness and left it behind us.

I walked and talked with other friends and acquaintances. It was wonderful to be with them in such a special environment. I felt extremely safe when I sat at meals and introduced myself to complete strangers. Three thousand of us, each with our own stories, shared a commitment to the same cause. Through shared dedication, we experienced warmth, compassion, and understanding as we walked the streets of southern California.

Along The Route

People lined the streets. We saw them on crowded sidewalks, in small groups or as single cheerleaders here and there. Drivers of all types of vehicles; cars, vans, trucks, buses, and motor cycles, honked their horns with gusto, waving and yelling, "You go girl!" Of course, that cheer was also for the men in our 3,000 plus cavalcade of walkers. It was amazing to see and hear all of those people cheering us on. I felt their intense wish for a cure for breast cancer. All of us were on track. Their encouragement kept us placing one-step in front of the other, in spite of sore muscles, blistered feet, and tired bodies.

On Friday, Day One, students from an entire elementary school were outdoors waiting to cheer us on. Each child held a sign, their own works of art, decorated with pink ribbons and words of encouragement. They held out their hands in the "high-five" position as we passed, which we returned with delight.

We stopped to take a picture and the children yelled,"I want to stand by you," as though we were celebrities.

Saturday we walked through a residential area. A man and three little girls waited in his driveway with "Free Cake and Lemonade for walkers!" He had thirty huge sheet cakes! The three girls, all under age ten, handed us pieces of wonderful chocolate cake with tons of frosting. What a treat!

Then they insisted we have lemonade because, as they said, "The cake may make you thirsty."

There were people who followed us all along the route. We saw the same cheerleaders repeatedly at different points throughout all three days.

We met innumerable people dedicated to the cause. A teenage girl pushed her mother in a wheel chair for the entire sixty miles, even through the woods, on bumpy trails. A woman who was being treated for cancer, walked ten miles on Saturday, left the event to go in for her chemotherapy treatment, and came back on Sunday for another ten miles. Another truly amazing person was a young woman who did the entire sixty miles on crutches because she had broken her foot the week before the walk and did not want to let down her supporters.

The crewmembers were awesome. They gave us snacks, power drinks, water; they sang songs, cheered, and performed antics to make us laugh. One crewmember asked the man who made evening announcements to mention that her son graduated on Saturday.

He said, "I can't do that. The announcements must be related to the walk."

She said, "Believe me, it is!" Her son missed his own high school graduation so he could support his mom by crewing for the 3 Day event.

We saw walkers with t-shirts designed to honor someone near to them who had succumbed to or were battling breast cancer. The shirts displayed pictures of mothers, sisters, daughters, and friends. Those displays of love brought tears to our eyes again & again.

The closing ceremony was incredible as we filled the street for the final mile into the Boston Common. I lost most of my voice because I yelled and cheered for my fellow walkers.

During those three days, my friend could not believe I could be so peppy at 6:00 a.m. I led cheers as we made our way through neighborhoods, not the least bit concerned about waking the neighbors. After all, we had already been up for hours. I wanted them to know we were there. Yet I was surprised at the number of people who were up early to say "thanks" as we passed by them.

I was taken by the overall spirit that surrounded all of us; walkers, crewmembers and cheering fans and supporters. I am grateful to have been a part of that incredible journey for such an important cause.

Karen's Thank You Letter

October 22, 2001

Dear Friends,

Today feels surreal. It juxtaposes the past three days of the best of humankind with the world reality of 9/11 and its aftermath, which demonstrated the worst of humankind. Please take a few minutes with me and revel in the best of humankind as I share with you the outcome of your generous financial and emotional support. Today follows three days of intense pain, pounding exhaustion, kindness, love, respect, and extreme admiration. Today is the day after my daughter, Jenny, and I completed the *Avon 3-Day* breast cancer walk, sixty-five miles from Santa Barbara to Malibu. Day one was to have been 22 miles; it was 26.3 miles. We did a marathon! Then woke up to do it again.

From last year's walk, I knew the kindness we would experience and the sheer exuberance that would sustain us, but Jenny was yet to know this. At the end of Day One, she reluctantly confessed that she thought she might be done. Everything hurt, really hurt. We decided not to make any decisions until the next morning, after we had an evening of putting ice on every body part possible. When 4:30 a.m. rolled around, we sluggishly put ourselves on automatic pilot; dressing in the pre-determined baggie-wrapped clothing, bandaging our feet, accessorizing with ID tags, pink ribbons, American flags and baseball caps.

In the foggy darkness, I asked, "How ya doin' kid?"

"So far so good," Jenny said.

That was it. Without actually reevaluating, we became part of the crunch of Ben Gay perfumed bodies softly singing *God Bless America* as we walked out the starting gate into Day 2.

We took care of each other, promising that we would listen to our bodies and if we needed to, we would end our walk. But the frequent rest stops set up for the walkers turned out to be goal markers for Jenny and me. We kept saying, "the next stop is only 1.8 miles, then 2.4 miles." In the totality of 65 miles, 2.4 was doable. Section after section after section brought us into Malibu. At least one-half mile from the finish line, we spotted hundreds of cheering supporters lining the Pacific Coast Highway. We interlaced fingers, looked at each other with glistening tears, hugged real tight, and then raised our hands to the cheering crowds. People wanted high fives, just to touch us, to connect to the cause and to the effort. Amidst happy faces, cheers, and sometimes shouts but often whispered words of thanks, there was Liz! Hers was the face that kissed us good bye in Santa Barbara three days earlier; hers was the first face, already wet with tears that kissed us hello in Malibu. Jumping from the crowd with outstretched arms, she grabbed us close. RD was easy to spot above the crowd, smiling, waiting his turn to scoop up Jenny. And there was my husband, wonderfully characteristic of him, quietly standing to the side, wearing a huge grin.

I am flooded with the journey's memories. The aching sadness when Jenny and I wrote messages on the Memory Banner to my mom and all the survivors we personally know; the quiet smile that surprised me each morning as I gently kissed the picture of Melanie and Elaine. Why the smile? Because as Melanie valiantly battled cancer, she gave me the warm gift of being more appreciative of each and every day.

And I gain strength from Elaine's words when I recall her saying about Melanie, "My final act as her mother is to make this passage as beautiful as possible for her."

I thank them for inviting me into their lives.

My thoughts shift to Mother-Daughter teams. We passed a seventeen year old girl who was adolescently cranky, giving her mom "those looks" with rolling eyes. Jenny quietly told her the girl's mother not to worry, that she and her daughter would be best friends in about five years. I smiled, as my heart overflowed with love for my daughter.

One daughter was to have flown in from Michigan but the events of September 11th interfered with their plan. Her mom did the walk without her, but not alone. She missed her daughter at her side but welcomed the friendship extended by 3,100 others.

A son, walking with his mother, wondered why so few guys were doing the walk; hadn't they discovered that it was a place to meet great women? On Day 2 his knees were talking. By Day 3 they were wrapped and he was limping. Determination had replaced joviality. He and his mom fell silent for the final miles into Malibu. But, most importantly, they began together and finished together.

We found a lost dog that a walker named "Avon." If the owner was not located, the walker who named her would adopt the friendly animal.

Then I saw Marge, the woman I met last year when I stopped to help an injured walker. The three of us finished the walk together in the drenching rain. I was amazed to find her this year among thousands of women! We hugged like long lost friends, which we were.

Two survivors, who were part of our group last year, surprised me on Day 2. They were on the side of the road, waving a giant neon yellow sign with my name on it! Instant prolonged hugs and tears! I tried to tell them how much it meant that they came out for me and that we actually found each other! They knew the pain, the intensity of the commitment, the difference each mile could make in their lives. Their words of thanks became a mantra for me as Day 3 loomed ominously ahead. Their joyful and grateful faces sustained me over and over again. How loved I felt!

After reaching the finish line and the visitors shuffled into seats in the bleachers for the closing ceremonies, Jenny and I were alone for a moment. Our tight, sustained hug, sobbing, looking at each other with renewed respect, and not letting go until the tears, for the moment, were spent. Why were we crying? The expression of pent up anxiety, from not just the three days of walking but also the weeks of training, and anticipating the pain and exhaustion. The sense of relief we felt, the joy of having completed such a huge goal, was almost overwhelming. It was all about the knowledge that someone was going to live because we walked.

There were sad stories of pain and heroic stories of courage. I vividly recall the face of a thirty-year old man saying that in a few days his blisters would be gone but the men and women with cancer would still have their tumors and their pain would not be gone.

"I can't stop crying," he told me. "I can't stop crying".

The night before we left for Santa Barbara, Jenny laid a note on my pillow attached to her check, made out to my Avon pledge account. The note said, "Because WE can." I walked for her; she walked for me. We walked for you, for your mothers, sisters, daughters, granddaughters, wives, and the men in their lives. Breast cancer kills men, too.

I feel blessed, grateful, and sustained. Thanks to each of you for your encouragement, praise, and money. Your generous pledges allowed me to have this intensely emotional, uplifting experience. Please know that your involvement also connected you to a bigger purpose, that of saving lives and finding a cure for breast cancer disease.

To anyone who wants to experience the event by walking, crewing, or volunteering, I want to say that I know you can give yourself a gift; you will earn your own confidence, knowing that you can satisfy a physical and emotional commitment that will make a real difference. Some mom will get to raise her kids because you are part of this.

Please remember that my ability to do this began with a significant weight loss, maintained now for over a year. For this, I continue to thank my supporters, my close friends and my family, who understand the lifetime commitment it requires and the changes they have tolerated in their lives to make my life work. The training for this event began not by counting miles, but by counting houses; how many houses could I walk past and still make it back home? Houses became blocks, blocks became miles. You, too, can reach your personal goals. Just respect yourself enough to make a plan that starts with tiny steps. They add up, just like the 2.4 miles plus the 1.8 miles added up to sixty-five miles. Amazing, huh?

My love and gratitude to each of you,

Karen

Conclusion

Life is a journey. We encounter joy and trials along the way. Caring for another person in need is an honor, even though it may be a difficult ordeal. He or she may be a close loved one, a friend, or someone with whom we crossed paths for a brief time. Regardless, the experience allows us a connection with humanity in a way that we feel deep within our souls.

One small act of kindness or a commitment of whole-hearted, time-consuming, loving involvement with a person with disease or disability opens a door for us to give a part of ourselves. Gifts of love and compassion are treasures to the recipient and bring joy to the giver.

Philosophers, religious and spiritual leaders, and those of us who traveled the road as caregivers, all share one of life's great blessings, that of love and compassion for one another.

The journey may be trying and, at times, extremely difficult. However, the human and spiritual connection we experience extends beyond our normal expectations. We discover it is true that **caregivers are angels without wings.**

Caregivers' Checklists

"I accept that I cannot change the winds but I can help trim the sails."

—Anonymous Caregiver

The first thing to discover, as a caregiver, is the truth in the above quote. You cannot be a "fixer" but you can make your loved one's journey smoother, helping navigate through the waves on the rough seas encountered with disease. The following checklists are suggestions, ideas, and recommendations that may ease your journey.

Primary and "Solo" Caregivers

The following checklists focus on tips for those who are primary/main caregivers for an ailing person. The suggestions are also directed towards patients who "go it alone," as their own primary caregiver. Circle those that are appropriate for you and review the list frequently, implementing suggestions that will ease your travels along the caregiver's path.

- Critical: Ask for help. Do not try to be Superman or Superwoman.

- Realize that your daily life has changed. It is doubtful that you will be able to stay on top of all you did before; let those things go; and do not feel guilty.

- Establish a hotline. Ask one or two friends to be key people whom you may contact when you need help. Then give them names of people you know would like to help so they can establish a phone tree. They will probably add other friend's names to the list.

- Delegate tasks to those who are willing to help: meal preparation, driving your patient to appointments, transporting children to their activities, picking up prescriptions…see the Occasional Caregivers' Checklist for additional suggestions.

178

- Make time for yourself!

- Relax: go to lunch with a friend, visit the art museum, ride your bike, walk, write in your journal, sip a cup of tea, listen to the birds sing, listen to music, and pursue your hobby.

- Emotionally drained? Find someone to talk with, vent your frustrations and feelings, cry, do something active to release anger, replace negative feelings with positive ones. Mentally, put your self in your favorite place.

- Manage your stress: Take deep breaths and exhale strongly to feel renewed energy; plan ahead but allow flexibility in your schedule; set priorities; do something that is not at all related to disease.

- Maintain your own health: Prepare food that is nutritious and easy to pull from the freezer and heat; exercise, get plenty of physical activity; rest, even if it is only stretching out on the couch for thirty minutes every afternoon; pursue activities that leave you feeling energized.

- Knowledge is power. Ask health care professionals what to expect regarding the disease, physical, and behavioral changes. Search the internet. Contact specific disease related organizations that can provide appropriate information and answer your questions.

- Join a support group! You need to talk about what is happening. Carrying the weight alone can become overwhelming.

Self-Advocates: Going Solo

- Ask your health-care professionals all the questions that enter your mind. Make notes between appointments.

- Jot down information you gain during your medical appointments.

- Search the internet for knowledge about your disease and care.

- Contact people who might help you work insurance issues.

- Join a support group!

- Review the checklist for primary caregivers and you!

- Remember that there are numerous sources of support: disease related groups, church members, neighbors, friends, organizations to which you have belonged. Just ask! People do want to help.

Hints on Helping Your Patient

- Respect his or her perspectives of the situation, even if they are different from yours.

- Project a positive attitude; view the glass as half full. A positive attitude is contagious. But don't be "gushy" or "phony." Be yourself!

- Be in the moment when you are with your friend or loved one. Stay tuned to their feelings and thoughts.

- Talk about normal life. They receive enough "I'm so sorry to hear…"

- Be a good listener. Let your patient talk about his or her concerns.

- Keep in mind that he or she may be cranky because they are feeling so poorly. Do not take it personally and try to bear with them. However, if they become too demanding, tell them you are becoming overwhelmed, and ask them to understand you are doing all you can.

- Accompany him to medical appointments. You can be an extra set of ears, take notes, and ask questions.

- Use the power of touch. Touch can enhance the healing process, and it certainly is comforting. Hug your loved one, hold hands, gently massage her arms, wash his hair, help him shave, give her a manicure, brush her hair. Put your arm around her or his shoulders.

- Look into his or her eyes when you speak. The connection is amazing.

- Quietly sit with your patient. Just being together, not saying a word, is an expression of love and a gift of caring.

- Divert your loved one's attention from their problems. Do things together: watch a movie (especially comedies), play a game, work a puzzle, listen to music, look at family pictures, or work on crafts. The two of you might build a model airplane, create a scrapbook, or make greeting cards. Being creative is an uplifting experience, especially when one is ill.

- Be playful. Have fun together, whether it is playing a game of checkers or taking a stroll in the park. Play makes people feel joyful.

- Give him or her something to anticipate. Plan an outing: visit the zoo, go to the theater, have a picnic.

- Celebrate everything! Have a party, invite a few friends. Decorate with balloons and streamers. Celebrate birthdays, holidays, hearing a child laugh, or seeing the first robin in spring.

Children and Teenagers Who are Caregivers

As a child or teenager, you may feel like there is not much you can do to help your loved one. Believe me, your love will shine through to your loved one by the small and major acts of kindness. Here are some suggestions made by young people in your position. Circle the ones you could do to be helpful.

- Draw pictures that he or she can hang in their room.

- Sing songs for your loved one, but ask first.

- Put on a short show. You could dance, sing, tell stories, or create a puppet show.

- Write a letter about what you are doing in school, scouts, gymnastics, baseball, dance class, football, or how you like skateboarding.

- Read or write poetry to your loved one.

- Help make meals.

- Make cards for your loved one.

- Sweep the kitchen floor.

- Keep your room clean.

Especially for Teenagers

- Talk with your loved one. Share what you are doing at school and in your activities, Tell her or him about what you and your friends are doing.

- Listen to music together.

- Watch a televised sporting event together.

- Talk about books, especially those that cover topics in which you are both interested.

- Prepare meals for your family.

- Help around the house: clean the kitchen, make the beds, dust, vacuum, do the laundry.

- Baby sit for the ill person or caregiver's children. Give them a break.

- Mow the lawn, shovel snow.

- If you have your driver's license, run errands or take your loved one to medical appointments. Take your loved one to the park or a movie, if they feel up to it.

- IMPORTANT! If you are asked to do a chore that you are not confident you can handle, simply ask how to go about accomplishing the task. There is no need to be up-tight; after all, we all continue to learn as we grow through life.

- REMEMBER that you, too, may need a break to see your friends or do something you enjoy. Ask your parents if you can schedule time for your activities.

Occasional Caregivers

Each act of kindness is meaningful. If you are wondering just how you can help your sick friend or their caregiver, consider the following suggestions. Circle those you or other friends could do for the patient or their family.

General

- Do not hesitate because you feel like you may be in the way. Ask what you can do.

On-Call

- Try to be available when needed

- Involve your friends in your compassionate mission. Create a phone tree to be employed when help is needed.

Help At Their Home

- Clean the kitchen

- Vacuum floors

- Dust

- Fold laundry

- Prepare meals, give gift certificates for meals to be delivered

- Share a ready to eat meal

Errands

- Grocery shop, pick up prescriptions at the pharmacy or books at the library, buy postage stamps

Relieve The Primary Caregiver

- Give the main caregiver a break. Stay with the patient so the caregiver can get out for a while.

- Take the primary caregiver to lunch or a movie

Phone, E-Mail, Cards, Surprises

- Leave phone messages such as, "Calling just to let you know I'm thinking of you. No need to return my call."

- Give emotional support through phone conversations

- E-mail messages and jokes

- Mail "thinking of you" notes or cards

Paper Work

- Write checks to pay bills so the patient only needs to add their signature

- Sort incoming mail (unopened, unless asked to remove the contents from the envelopes) by categories, i.e. bills, first class, catalogs, junk mail

Visit

- Converse about normal life

- Discuss topics that interest the patient

- Reminisce about good times

- Laugh and cry together

- Be in the moment

- Watch movies, listen to music

- Read a book aloud

- Help with crafts or hobbies

- Write letters or e-mails to your patients friends; let him or her dictate the message

- Celebrate anything and everything

- Bring balloons or flowers

For the Children in the Family

- Give the children a lot of attention

- Take them to a movie

- Have them spend the night at your home

- Help with homework

- Chauffeur children to activities

- Attend a cub scout or brownie meeting with the children

- If one of the parents cannot meet with the teacher, volunteer to do so

Religious or Spiritual

- Start a prayer chain

- Pray or meditate together

- Perform rituals

Medical

- Drive the patient to medical appointments

- Schedule appointments

- Research relative information

- Visit with patient during chemo treatments

- Set up spread sheet to be used for medical information

Long Distance Caregivers

Geographic distance does not need to be an overwhelming barrier when you have a friend or loved one struggling with disease. Long distance caregivers provided the following tips on how to extend your support across the miles.

- Stay in touch by phone. Talk about day to day happenings, laugh and cry together, listen to favorite music together (yes, even while on the phone), surprise your patient by having a mutual friend join in on your conversation.

- Provide emotional support. Listen to what he or she is feeling and thinking, including their fears and problems. Avoid saying, "Don't worry, everything will be okay."

- Talk about good times you have shared.

- Send e-mail messages. Instant message one another.

- E-mail funny stories and greeting cards.

- Transmit jokes electronically.

- Use United States Postal Service.

- Send notes and cards.

- Send small gifts: books, magazines, games or small craft projects, movie rental gift certificates, musical CDs.

- Have balloons or flowers delivered.

- Once a week, mail a card. Anticipation of the next card in a series can be uplifting.

- Find a reasonable airfare or make a road trip. Surprise your friend by visiting.

APPENDIX

I encourage you to search the web or speak with health care professionals regarding resources that may be specific to your needs. However, the following organizations are a few of the numerous resources available to caregivers. Although the contact information has been verified, the websites or phone numbers may change in the future.

Caregiver Websites

- www.caregiver.com

- Caregiver Connection http://www.caressentials.com/cconnect.htm

- Caregiver Online (sponsored as a free service by Family Caregiver Alliance)
  http://www.caregiver.org/online_sptgroup.html
  or send e-mail to CAREGIVER-ONLINE@PEACH.EASE.LSOFT.COM

- National Family Caregivers Association
  www.nfcacares.org

Disease-Related Organization Websites

- **American Heart Association**
  www.americanheart.org

- American Stroke Association
  www.strokeassociation.org

- Diabetes
  www.diabetes.org

- Leukemia
  http://www.leukemia-lymphoma.org

- Multiple Sclerosis
  www.mswatch.com

- Prostate Cancer
  http://www.pcacoalition.org

- Help parents and children with cancer
  http://www.candlelighters.org

- Help children facing cancer within the family http://www.kidscope.org
  http://www.kidskonnected.org

Disease-Related Organization Phone Numbers

- The American Cancer Society
  1-800-ACS-2345

- American Diabetes Association
  1-800-232-3472

- American Heart Association
  1-800-AHA-USA1

- Arthritis Foundation
  1-800-965-7540

- National Stroke Association
  1-800-STROKES

- Susan G. Komen Breast Cancer Foundation
  1-800-I'M AWARE

- (National Cancer Institute)
  NCI/Cancer Information Service
  1-800-4CANCER

- Cancer
  1-800-4cancer

About the Author

Peg Crandall is a cancer survivor and an on-going caregiver for a myriad of people fallen victim to disease. She has volunteered at the Nevada Cancer Center, Susan G. Komen Race for the Cure, and the American Cancer Society Relay for Life where she spoke to caregivers and cancer patients. She was active in a cancer support group, and participated as a walker and crewmember in two Avon 3-Day events for breast cancer.

The inspiration for *Caregivers: Angels without Wings* came to Peg after she and her sister, both diagnosed with breast cancer, received an outpouring of love and support from friends and family. However, this book is not limited to any specific disease because she chose to present caregivers' universal experiences, regardless of the physical disabilities encountered by their loved ones. Gathering stories and words of wisdom for this book, Peg interviewed more than fifty people and talked with innumerable others who have been caregivers or recipients of caregivers' love and support.

She has published magazine and newspaper articles. Her stirring story about the wonders of people bonding together in support of a health-related cause was the highlight of a Nevada Woman Magazine issue.

She is a graduate of Drury University and holds a Masters Degree from Webster University. Peg resides with her husband, Marv, in Aurora, Colorado. She is passionate about supporting caregivers and speaks to groups who relate to this topic.

Peg Crandall can be reached by e-mail: caregiversangelswithoutwings@yahoo.com

0-595-32660-9